HEALTHY
BODY

To Ros!
Welcome
to the Shredder
family :)

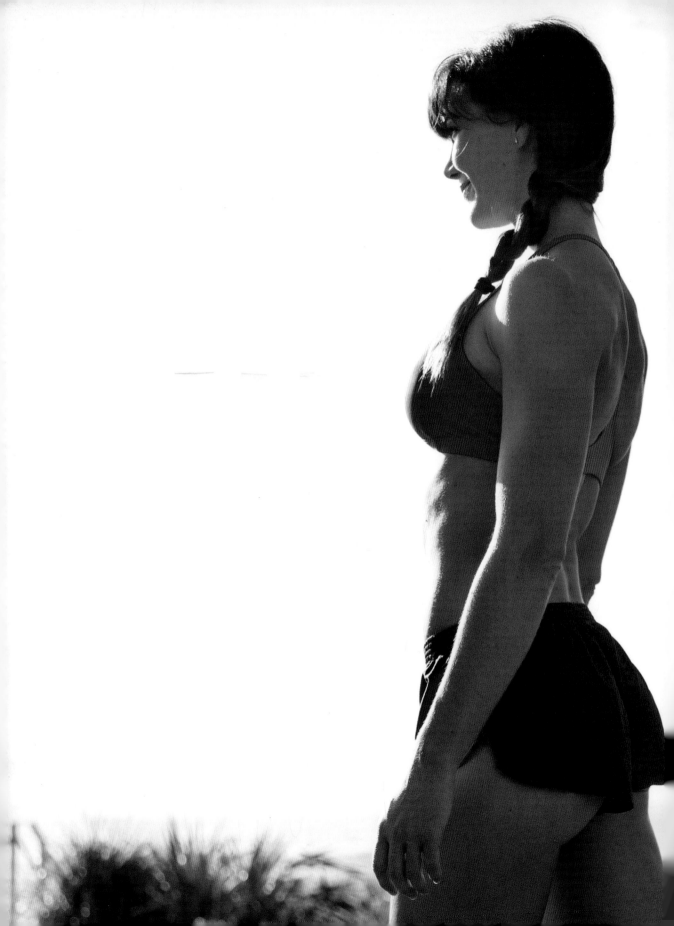

Healthy Living Series

HEALTHY
BODY

*balance your hormones
and shred fat for life*

SALLY MATTERSON

ROCKPOOL
PUBLISHING

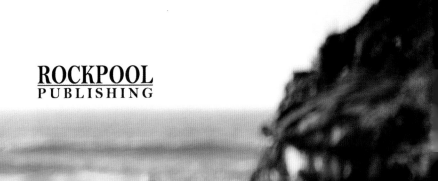

I would like to thank my family for supporting me on this journey and always encouraging me to pursue my dreams, whatever it takes.

To my beautiful fur baby, Bambi, who has been a very cute and cuddly distraction. Thanks for all those much-needed puppy cuddles and kisses along the way.

And last, but definitely not least, to the man upstairs. My God. Thank you for always blessing me with opportunities to do amazing positive things in this world and for always having my back in the hard times. My faith in you has got me through many a tough moment. I have always felt your presence helping me get to the end of this project and as a result, hundreds if not thousands of people will have the tools to get stronger, leaner and gain better health. Can I get an amen to that!

Yours in health and fitness,

Sally Matterson

A Rockpool book
PO Box 252
Summer Hill NSW 2103
rockpoolpublishing.com.au
facebook.com/RockpoolPublishing
ISBN 9781925017526 (pbk.)
Text © 2015 Sally Matterson
Photographs © 2015 Rockpool Publishing

Editor: Megan English
Designer: Stan Lamond
Photographer (exercises): Natalie Roser
Photographer (food): Brent Parker Jones
Food stylist: Lee Blaylock
Chef: Mark Hockenull
Kitchen prep chef: Nick Tanti
Photographs (pages 14, 19, 90): Shutterstock
Printed and bound in China

10 9 8 7 6 5 4 3 2 1

Disclaimer

Healthy body is designed to help you shred body fat by eating the way your body was supposed to and is supported by specific exercise work-outs.

Readers are responsible for their own choices in regard to their health and the implementation of any material found in *Healthy body*.

The author and publisher are not medical practitioners. Their intent is to offer health-related information. As such, they do not prescribe that any of the material contained herein be used for the diagnosis, treatment or prescription of any illness or medical condition. If this is required, it is recommended that you consult the appropriate health professionals. In addition, medical clearance is recommended for those participants with injuries and illnesses that may affect their training.

contents

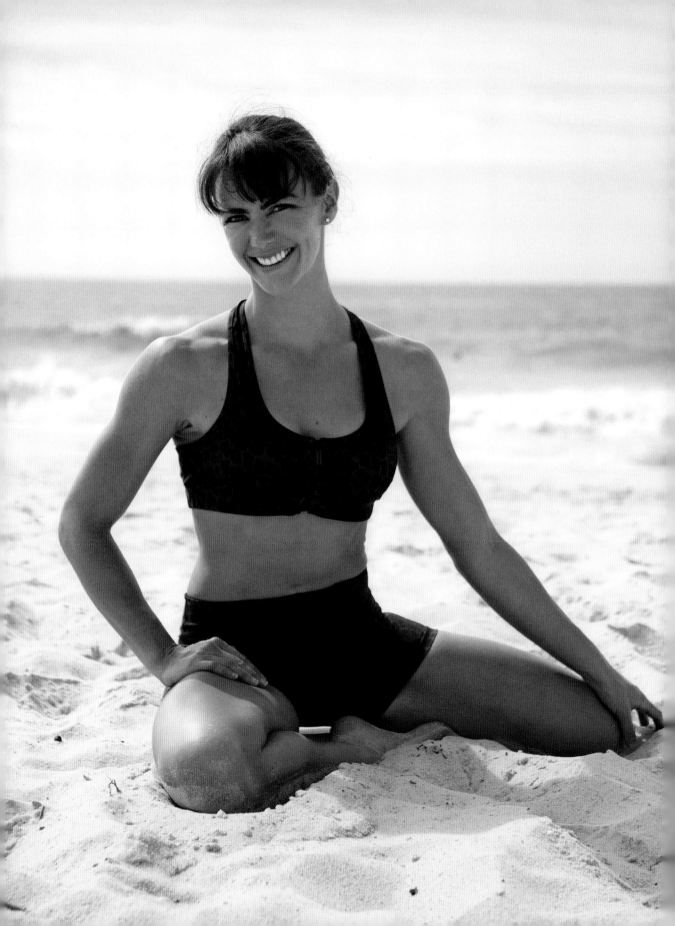

a message
from the
author

'When you're fit, you're happy.'

Welcome.

Healthy body gives you the tools to get your body into the best condition of your life! Not only will you look better, but you will feel amazing as you strip body fat and eat the way your body was supposed to. I call this process shredding – and I know it works, firsthand.

After leading a fast-paced lifestyle in the fashion industry for many years, I desperately needed to focus on my health. My body type was what you might call skinny fat – the type that looks okay in clothes, but jiggles when you run or walk. I ate very little and when I did, it was usually soya crisps and a can of Coke topped off with a couple of ciggies before I headed back to my desk. Shocking, I know!

So even though I was thin, I was very unhealthy. As a result, I felt terrible most of the time – frail, weak and battling a constant brain fog. I was miserable and depressed, too. But the reality of my unhealthy lifestyle only really hit me when my dad collapsed from a heart condition. He needed surgery, which fortunately saved his life, but his health crisis had a huge impact on me. I knew that if I didn't change my own unhealthy lifestyle, I was heading down the same road. I needed to take control of my health – straight away.

It was at this point that I felt courageous enough to take my first baby step toward achieving my fitness goals and join a health club. That was over 12 years ago and I have never looked back! Best of all, when I finally got fit, I got happy. And when I took control of my health, my inner strength increased, too.

Needless to say, it has been an amazing journey. I have tried several methods of training in my time, and found this to be the most effective. It is about training smarter, not harder – training and eating right to balance your hormones, rather than throw them out of whack.

I know just how hard and frustrating getting fit and losing body fat can be. I have tried several fads in my time! Low carb, high carb, low calorie, interval training, marathons (my knees are screaming at the thought of it, even now!), spin classes, CrossFit, BodyPump ... you name it, I've tried it.

But over the last seven years, I have really nailed what I would call the smartest way to stay lean for life and it doesn't involve eating like a bodybuilder or restricting calories. It doesn't mean endless hours at the gym or running marathons to get in shape, either. It is, first and foremost, about knowing your body and how to eat right for it.

By knowing your body, I mean learning how your body functions hormonally and how this affects your health, your wellbeing and your ability to lose fat. Once you understand the hormonal rules that govern your body, you will become the master of your physique, shred fat and finally be in control of your own body.

I came to this understanding through years of research and by obtaining my qualifications as a Poliquin® BioSignature practitioner – the underpinning to all my work and the fabulous results my clients (affectionately known as shredders!) are able to achieve. I have written this book to share this knowledge with you. It is my hope that by understanding the intricate details of your hormones in a simple, easy-to-understand way, you can create your own, ultimate healthy body, too.

One of the most empowering things you can ever do for yourself, and for the people around you, is to make the right choices for your body and improve your overall lifestyle. Remember, you have full control over what goes in your mouth and how hard you train. You have the power to change and turn your dreams into reality. Through loving and respecting yourself and your body, you can eliminate old habits, release toxic things from your life and allow new, life-changing, positive stuff into your world.

A healthy body makes for a healthy mind and can improve every aspect of your existence. By putting my health first, I have at last found true happiness and peace in my life. I have proved this to myself over and over, and now it is your turn.

So shredders, let's get started!

POLIQUIN® BIOSIGNATURE

Poliquin® BioSignature Modulation is a cutting-edge, non-invasive fat loss method. It is a method based on the correlation between body fat distribution and possible hormonal imbalances. Hormonal imbalances are often the culprit of stubborn body fat storage and other health concerns such as poor sleep, low energy, impaired cognitive function, and more. Poliquin® BioSignature Modulation focuses on addressing these imbalances to improve body composition and wellbeing.

Through specific body fat measurements and client assessment, Poliquin® BioSignature practitioners recommend an individualised program of nutrition, supplementation, and lifestyle modifications to lose stubborn body fat and achieve wellness.

To be clear, Poliquin® BioSignature Modulation is not spot reduction, however hormonal fat gain is spot gaining. Using the techniques of Poliquin® BioSignature can help balance your chemistry in order to repartition fat stores.

You will also see improvements in many other areas of your life, too. Participants commonly report increased mental clarity, improved quality of sleep, higher energy levels and better moods. You can achieve all of this without unsafe fat-loss pills, hours of aerobic work, or unhealthy diet plans by simply using the principles contained within *Healthy body*.

For an even better understanding of the concepts within this book or for information specific to your body and lifestyle, I would recommend seeking the advice of a Poliquin® BioSignature practitioner. To start, visit www.poliquingroup.com and search for practitioner near you who will be able to do a one-on-one analysis. I would strongly recommend this if you are serious about finding out more about your hormones and body fat composition.

Let's go, shredders!

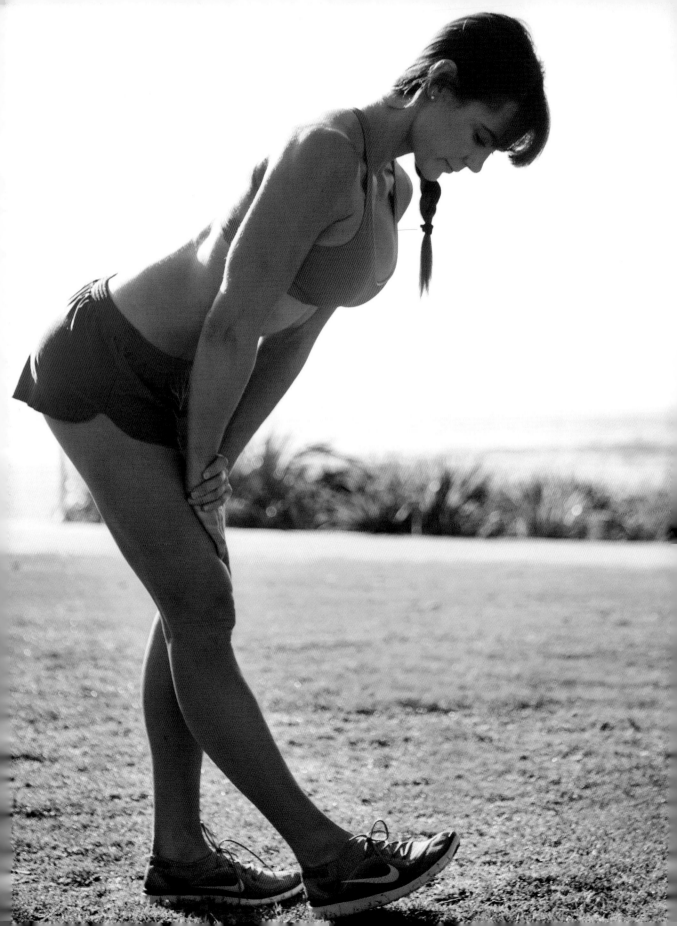

shred body fat *by* balancing your hormones

'First and foremost, I want to educate people because I believe it will create lifelong change.'

A lot of diet and weight-loss books will tell you if you eat this and train like that you will get this result. What a lot fail to do is tell you why you are doing it.

Over years spent training clients, I have noticed that once they understand *why* they are doing something, they can change it for life instead of just doing it because I say so or to get a quick-fix result.

First and foremost, I want to educate people because I believe it will create *lifelong* change. I am not about quick fixes or fast and often dangerous approaches. I want to give sound advice based on what I know about how supplementation, training and nutrition work together to help significantly reduce body fat.

I want to give sound advice based on what I know about how supplementation, training and nutrition work together to help significantly reduce body fat.

A lot of it comes down to understanding key hormones and how they change in your body as you age, as well as the major role diet and lifestyle play in this process. To make it really simple, I focus on the four key areas in the body where fat is stored depending on possible hormonal imbalances:

- jelly-belly fat (surrounding the navel)
- love handles and/or back fat
- pear-shaped body and/or jelly legs
- bat-wing arms and/or upper chest fat (surrounding the heart).

If you tend to store body fat everywhere, I have some solutions for you, too. But first, following is a run-down on each of the body types listed above as well as the hormone responsible and a possible solution to help control further imbalances in the body.

Sals QUICK TIP

To a degree, our genetic make-up does dictate hormonal levels in the body, but a lot can be controlled by lifestyle and good nutrition.

JELLY-BELLY FAT

Doesn't sound very appealing, does it! We all know what jelly belly looks, and feels, like! It is that uncomfortable fat gain predominantly around the belly-button area that doesn't seem to affect the rest of your body, so you may still have relatively slim arms and legs.

Hormone responsible: cortisol

Cortisol is a hormone released by the cortex (the outer portion) of the adrenal gland when a person is under stress. It can be so destructive that cortisol levels are now considered a biological marker of suicide risk. Excess or continued high levels of cortisol contributes greatly to body-fat storage around the navel area.

Why does cortisol increase weight in this area?

When you are stressed, your body over-produces the hormone cortisol. As a result, your body holds on to fat. Since there are more cortisol receptors in the abdomen, when we are stressed, the body tends to hold on to fat in this area.

This unhealthy visceral fat (the fat surrounding your internal organs), can also increase inflammation and insulin resistance in the body, further increasing body fat and creating a vicious cycle of fat production throughout the whole body. The risk of developing adrenal fatigue and chronic fatigue as a result is also increased.

Solution

Stress less! Easier said than done sometimes, but worth the effort. Focus on adopting regular sleeping patterns, taking up light activities, meditating, connecting with others and new activities or seek professional help if required.

If stress is unavoidable, try supplementing with magnesium. Taken in the evening, this will act as a cortisol blocker and help relax the body, relieving anxiety, too. I suggest starting with a modest dose of 300-600 mg a day, increasing up to 4000 mg a day if symptoms of stress and sleeplessness are still present.

Sals QUICK TIP . . . .

Many endurance athletes are at risk of increased cortisol levels due to excessive cardiovascular exercise. The best way to increase cardiovascular fitness with minimal cortisol production is to train using shorter intervals and shorter sessions, combining weights and cardio-based exercise such as sprinting or skipping.

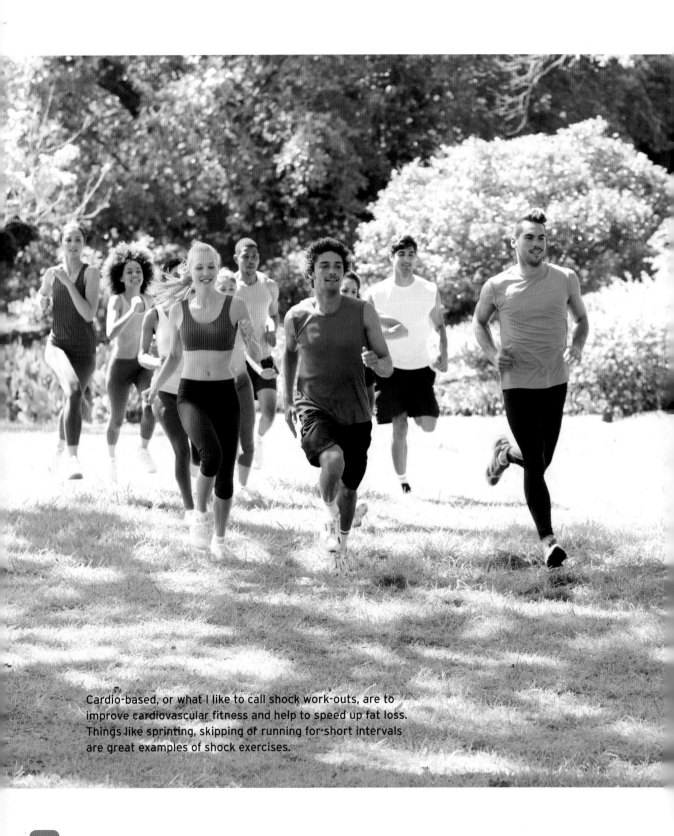

Cardio-based, or what I like to call shock work-outs, are to
improve cardiovascular fitness and help to speed up fat loss.
Things like sprinting, skipping or running for short intervals
are great examples of shock exercises.

healthy body: balance your hormones and shred fat for life

LOVE HANDLES AND/OR BACK FAT

Love handles, cute as they may sound, are unfortunately not very healthy. Those rolls of fat on your hips (also known as a muffin top), or on your back, have a lot to say about your health.

Hormone responsible: insulin

A major fuel-regulating hormone, insulin is secreted into the blood from the pancreas. Its function is to store and transport energy from carbohydrates (in the form of glucose) to the muscles for energy.

Why does insulin increase weight in this area?

Unfortunately, when we consume too many carbs, we produce too much insulin, which rather than being used for energy, gets stored as fat. Over time, this can cause insulin resistance, which means the body cannot tolerate carbs anymore. This is often reflected physically in fat distribution on the shoulder blades and the top of the hips, otherwise known as love handles.

Shoulder blade skinfold thickness is also directly associated with carbohydrate intolerance and research suggests that fat in this area may, in some cases, help identify risk of type 2 diabetes in pre-menopausal women.

Solution

Once the body becomes insulin resistant, it goes into a meltdown. This can be corrected by controlling carbohydrate intake in the diet and taking EPA-dominant, pharmaceutical-grade omega-3 fish oil, both of which can help increase your insulin sensitivity. In short, you will produce less insulin and when you do eat carbs, they will be used the way they should be – for energy!

PEAR-SHAPED BODY AND/OR JELLY LEGS

Yes, a pear-shaped body is beautiful and feminine – and sometimes this is our natural shape – but sometimes we can have too much of a good thing. Same with jelly legs. Enough said!

Hormone responsible: oestrogen

Secreted from the ovaries, oestrogen is the female sex hormone that regulates the female characteristics of the body such as reproduction, menstruation and menopause. However, excess oestrogen can also be ingested from our environment, causing havoc with our bodies and body fat composition.

Why does oestrogen increase weight in this area?

An imbalance in oestrogen levels can be caused by many different factors and will be specific to your lifestyle and age. However, one main cause that affects many women is the presence of xenoestrogens (or what we call oestrogen mimickers) from our environment (found in plastics, pesticides and parabens). These mimickers can latch on to existing receptors, which are predominantly found in the lower half of the body, causing fat to be stored in this area.

Solution

To rid excess oestrogen from the body and in turn lean out your legs, try and avoid or minimise the toxins or oestrogen mimickers from entering your body, while getting your body efficient at detoxing through the use of supplementation.

To reduce the effect of xenoestrogens from the environment, try to limit the toxic load on the body by:

- using glass or ceramic instead of plastic to eat or drink from
- choosing paraben-free products (check the ingredients list on your cosmetics, food products and pharmaceuticals)
- buying organic fruit and vegies
- washing produce thoroughly with water.

The kidneys, liver and gastrointestinal tract are all responsible for detoxing foreign oestrogens from the body, so it is important that they function well. To speed up the detoxification process and clean out trouble spots:

- ensure you drink lots of water
- increase your intake of cruciferous vegies containing sulforaphane and indoles (such as kale, brussels sprouts, spinach and cabbage).

We can also reduce the load on the body from xenoestrogens by supplementing our diet with:

- a pharmaceutical-grade multivitamin containing zinc and B-vitamins – to help metabolise foreign oestrogens from the body, particularly from the liver and kidneys.
- a probiotic and digestion support or HCL (hydrochloric acid, see below) – to support the gastrointestinal (GI) tract and help excrete oestrogens from the intestine.
- flaxseed lignans – a good, plant-based oestrogen, flaxseed can bind to oestrogen receptor sites before the nasty ones get there, inhibiting further production.

Sals QUICK TIP

HCL, or hydrochloric acid, is a good stomach acid. When taken orally, it can help break down foods, allowing vital vitamins and minerals to be absorbed. Some symptoms of low hydrochloric acid are belching, bloating, acid reflux after eating, indigestion, constipation and acne.

It is also worthwhile making sure that you are absorbing folic acid (B-vitamins) properly. Although not as accurate as a proper lab test, you can quickly test your absorption by performing the asparagus test. If your urine smells strong and repugnant after eating asparagus, chances are that you have a gene that will inhibit you processing B-vitamins, which is essential for detoxification.

BAT-WING ARMS AND/OR UPPER CHEST FAT

Bat wings, or bingo arms, are those dreaded folds of skin under the arms that wobble when you lift your arms. Luckily, like the fat that accumulates on the chest around the heart, sometimes called man boobs, there is something that can be done to help.

Hormone responsible: DHEA

Produced by your adrenal glands, DHEA (or dehydroepiandrosterone), is the largest raw material your body uses to produce other vital hormones, including testosterone in men and women.

Your body's natural production of DHEA varies widely with age. Very low levels are produced before puberty, with peak production in your late 20s or early 30s, followed by a steady decline in production with age.

Research is currently being undertaken into the anti-ageing properties of DHEA.

Why does DHEA increase weight in this area?

People with low DHEA have significantly lower levels of mid-arm muscle than those with normal levels of DHEA. Along with decreased muscle tone, they also have the dreaded arm wobble or bat-wing arm.

Another symptom of low DHEA is excess fat on the chest, also referred to as man boobs. This indicates that the male sex hormones (testosterone) are being converted to female sex hormones (oestrogen), rather than being utilised for muscle development and fat loss. In the male body, this is often referred to as aromatisation and is often present in males with a zinc deficiency.

> ## *Sal's* QUICK TIP
>
> When cortisol production is also high, especially for prolonged periods of time, your adrenals can wear out and DHEA production can suffer as well.
>
> Cortisol management will also ensure DHEA levels stay at their optimum.

Solution

As a long-term solution for fat loss, I recommend boosting DHEA levels naturally by taking up weight-bearing exercise like weight lifting and increasing your intake of protein. This will help the growth of lean muscle mass.

Low DHEA levels can also be linked to a zinc deficiency (as described above), so a pharmaceutical-grade zinc supplement or multivitamin can help restore zinc to appropriate levels in the body.

If necessary, a blood test from your GP can test your DHEA levels. You may be prescribed a DHEA supplement, which has been shown to significantly improve DHEA levels.

EVERYWHERE FAT

If you're storing fat everywhere, you know it. Your dress or clothes size is consistently going up and you just feel like your weight is out of control. The bad news is, increased weight increases your risk of diseases like type 2 diabetes, heart disease and obesity, to name a few. The good news is, this is not a necessary part of getting older. By simply improving your nutrition first and foremost, you can help restore balance to your hormones and lead a better quality of life.

Start by increasing the protein in your diet and decreasing the processed sugar and fat. This alone can significantly decrease the risk of lifestyle-related illnesses.

I also highly recommend a pharmaceutical-grade omega-3 fish oil. This alone will reduce inflammation and make your body more insulin sensitive. What that means is that when you eat carbohydrates, you will use the glycogen for energy, rather than store it as fat.

Sal's QUICK TIP ·

If you are very insulin resistant, you will find it hard to lose body fat and again, it can put you at a greater risk of type 2 diabetes. Seek professional help in the form of a certified medical practitioner.

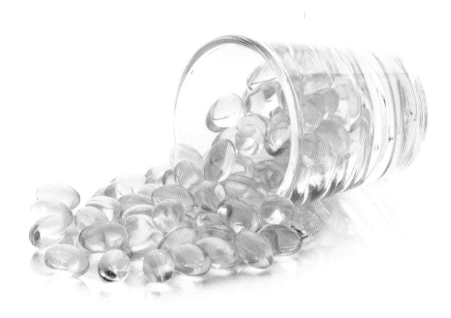

I highly recommend a pharmaceutical-grade omega-3 fish oil. This alone will reduce inflammation and make your body more insulin sensitive.

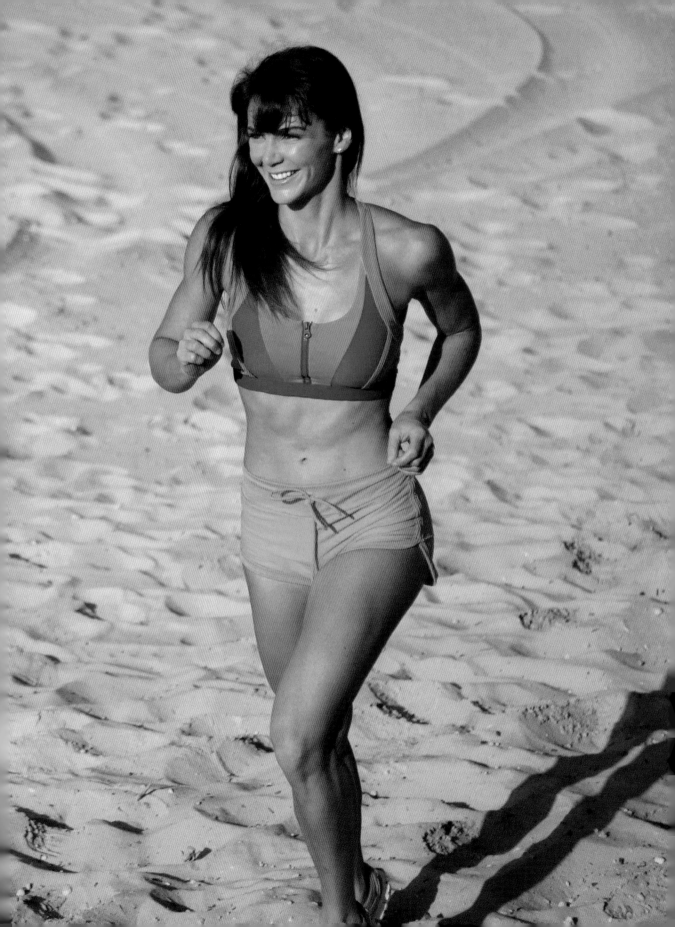

boost your metabolism *with* exercise

Let's go, shredders! A stronger, leaner and shapelier body is just around the corner ...

Weight-bearing exercise is essential for lean muscle development. The more lean muscle we have, the faster our metabolism. This will, in turn, burn fat faster. Let's go, shredders!

THE WEEKLY WORK-OUT SCHEDULE

The circuits below have been specifically designed to boost your metabolism while toning the body. If you are new to training, start with the three-day work-out, then move on to the five-day work-out after six weeks.

If, however, you have been exercising regularly, you can start with the five-day work-out straight away.

Both work-outs target specific muscle groups using weighted circuits. For maximum effectiveness, combine with a Shredder Shock Work-out (SSWO) to finish.

Sals QUICK TIP

The Shredder Shock Work-Outs (or SSWO) training sessions will also help those struggling to get their nutrition spot-on according to my guidelines. If you are diligent at following the meal plan, the weight-based training circuits should be more than adequate for fat loss.

I cannot stress how important intensity is to the work-out. Work quickly but effectively, maintaining a good and safe technique.

Equipment

To complete the work-outs, you'll need a few basic items (see image opposite):

- fitball
- dumbbells (3, 4 and 5 kg)
- weight plate or medicine ball (minimum 10 kg)
- step (such as Reebok, optional)
- skipping rope (optional).

Sals QUICK TIP

Shredder Shock Work-outs don't require any equipment and can be done inside or outside.

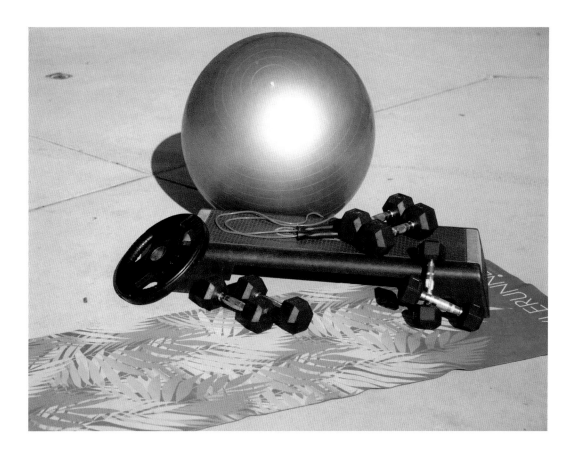

Completion

For every work-out, you complete two circuits, each with four stations.

First complete stations A1 to A4, four times through.

Then move from B1 to B4, four times through.

Follow this up with an SSWO and you'll really be sweating!

Repetitions (reps)

This is the repetition range at which you complete the exercises. For example, if the reps specified are 10, that means that you complete the exercise 10 times.

Sets

A set is a completed series of repetitions. For example, a completed round of 10 reps is one set.

So, if you're performing four sets, this would mean you complete a total of 40 reps in sets of 10, with a rest period after each set.

Tempo

Tempo refers to the timing of the exercise. The first number is the lowering (down) phase of the exercise, the second number indicates if a pause is required, the third number is the lifting (up) phase of the exercise and the fourth indicates if another pause is required. For example a tempo of 4010 indicates an up phase of 1, no pause, a down phase of 4 and no pause at the bottom.

Sal's QUICK TIP

Shredder Shock Work-outs don't include a tempo as you do them as fast as you can within the time allocated.

Rest

The rest is the transition period from one exercise to the next. So, if the rest period is 10 seconds, you've really only got enough time to move from the end of one exercise to the beginning of the next. These work-outs are designed to be intense, hence the typically short rest period.

Weight

The weight selection is based on personal strength and repetition range. Choose a weight that will bring the muscle to failure in the specified number of reps/sets. If the weight you've chosen doesn't bring you to failure after you've completed your sets, it's time to go heavier.

Sal's QUICK TIP

By failure, I mean that you are unable to do any more repetitions while maintaining correct form.

Schedule

If you are just starting out as a shredder, do the beginners' weekly work-out schedule consisting of three days of training and four days of rest. You can change which days you train, as long as all three training days are completed in the scheduled order.

For the advanced shredder, however, the weekly work-out schedule consists of five days of training and two days of rest. You can change which days you train, as long as all five training days are completed in the scheduled order. For example you could change to training on days 1 and 2, rest day 3, train days 4, 5 and 6, rest day 7.

Sal's QUICK TIP

When possible, days 1 and 2 are repeated on days 4 and 5 respectively because they are our big compound lifts or our big, fat-burning, calorie-busting exercises. They are also structured in such a way to give proportion to the body and develop muscle, which gives you a toned, muscular, fitness-model physique.

3-DAY BEGINNER SHREDDER weekly overview

Remember, you can change which days you train, as long as all three training days are completed in the scheduled order.

Day 1: Back and quads + SSWO 1 (optional)

Day 2: Shoulders, glutes and hamstrings + SSWO 2 (optional)

Day 3: Arms and abs + SSWO 3 (optional)

(Plus four days of rest.)

5-DAY ADVANCED SHREDDER weekly overview

Remember, you can change which days you train, as long as all five training days are completed in the scheduled order.

Day 1: Back and quads + SSWO 1 (optional)

Day 2: Shoulders, glutes and hamstrings + SSWO 2 (optional)

Day 3: Arms and abs + SSWO 3 (optional)

Day 4: Back and quads + SSWO 1 (optional)

Day 5: Shoulders, glutes and hamstrings + SSWO 2 (optional)

(Plus two days of rest.)

days 1 & 4

back and
quads
+ SSWO 1

First complete the four-station A circuits, four times
through. Then move through the four-station B circuits,
four times through.

Follow this up with SSWO 1, if desired, completing all the
As in the three-station circuit, then all the Bs, then all
the Cs in under 20 minutes or for time - that is, as fast
as you can!

A1

Bent over row with plate

Stand with feet hip distance apart.

Tip from the hip, making sure you load through the heels to ensure the glutes and hamstrings are taking on the load.

Draw the shoulders away from the ears and pull the plate in towards the navel while squeezing the shoulder blades together.

Lower the plate slowly for 4 seconds to your original position.

12, 4 sets, 4-0-1-0, 10 sec rest

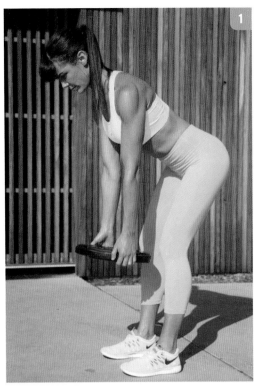

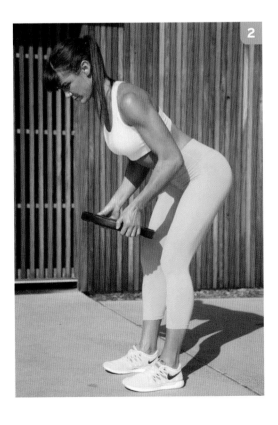

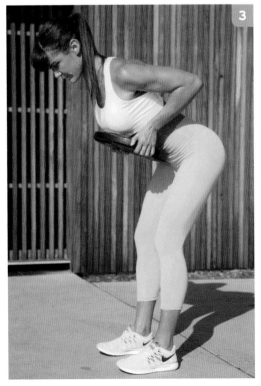

A2

Wide-stance squat with plate

Stand with feet wide apart and toes turned out at a slight angle.

Keeping the chest upright at all times, lower the body down for 4 seconds, keeping the weight through the heels and the focus on the glutes.

Drive up through the heels for 1 second, squeezing the glutes and returning to the original position.

15, 4 sets, 4-0-1-0, 10 sec rest

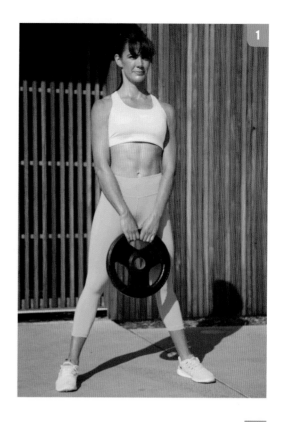

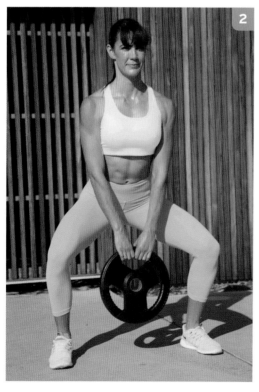

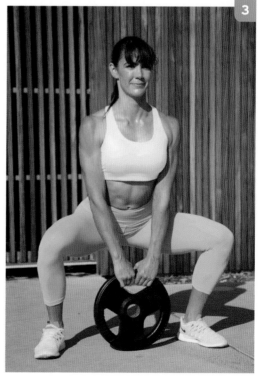

A3

Dumbbell bent-over row

Stand with feet hip distance apart.

Tip from the hip, making sure you load through the heels to ensure the glutes and hamstrings are taking the load.

Keeping the dumbbells close to the body, draw the shoulders away from the ears and row dumbbells up for 1 second while squeezing the shoulder blades together.

Lower down to the original position for 3 seconds.

20, 4 sets, 3-0-1-0, 10 sec rest

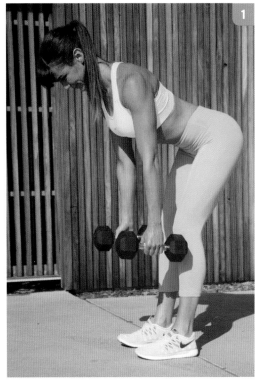

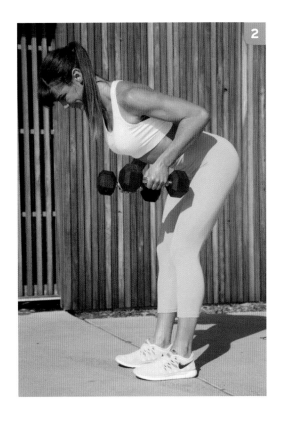

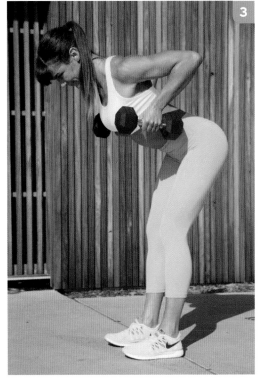

A4

Walking lunge

Place one foot (slightly turned out) in front of the other and lower or lunge down into the front heel for 2 seconds. Then drive up for 1 keeping the weight in the heel.

Switch feet and repeat until 20 repetitions are completed in total (ie 10 on each leg).

20, 4 sets, 2-0-1-0, 10 sec rest

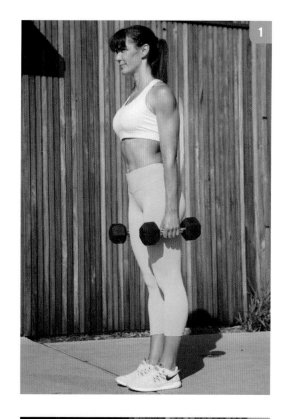

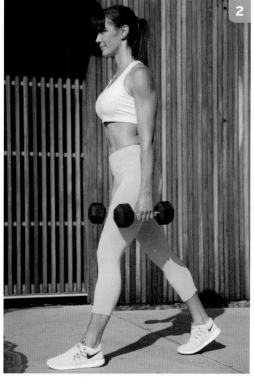

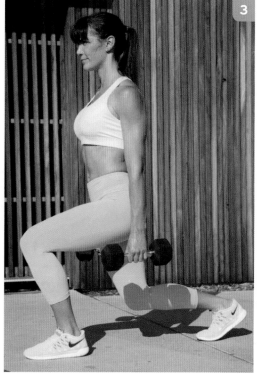

healthy body: balance your hormones and shred fat for life

B1

Dumbbells reverse fly

Stand feet hip distance apart.

Tip from the hip, making sure you load through the heels to ensure the glutes and hamstrings are taking on the load.

Draw the shoulder away from the ears and keep a slight bend at the elbow joint.

Bring the dumbbells up for 1 second, squeezing the back of the shoulder. Then lower down for 3 seconds, keeping the hands outside of the thighs.

12, 4 sets, 3-0-1-0, 10 sec rest

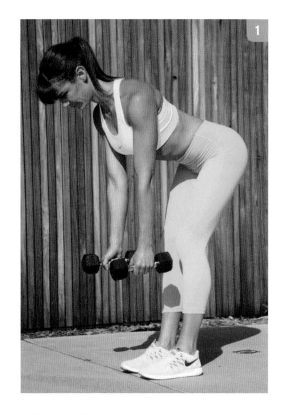

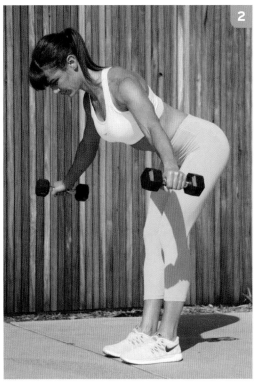

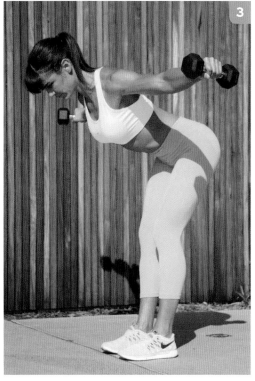

B2

Bench lunge

Elevate one leg onto the step or bench. Keep the hips in one line, turning the toe of the front leg out slowly.

Lower your body weight into the front leg for 4 seconds, focussing the weight into the heel. Squeeze the glutes on the way up for 1 second.

Repeat 12 times then switch legs.

12 each leg, 4 sets, 4-0-1-0, 10 sec rest

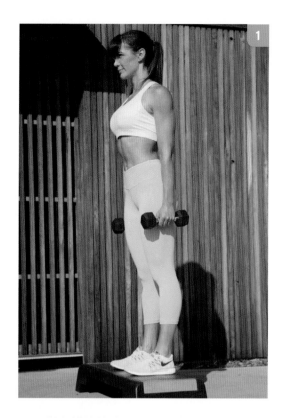

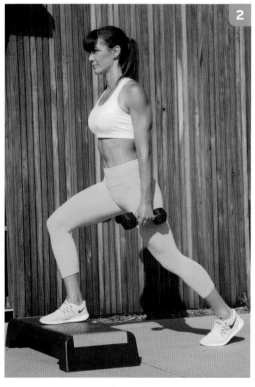

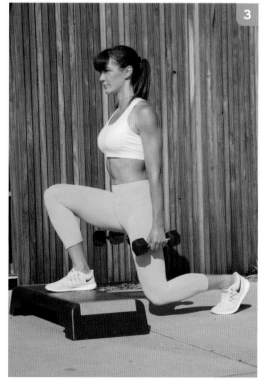

B3

Dumbbell external rotation

Taking the elbow into a 90-degree angle, bring the dumbbells up to shoulder height.

Rotate the shoulders, keeping the 90-degree angle at all times.

Lower the weights down for 2 seconds to the original starting position.

20, 4 sets, 2-0-1-0, 10 sec rest

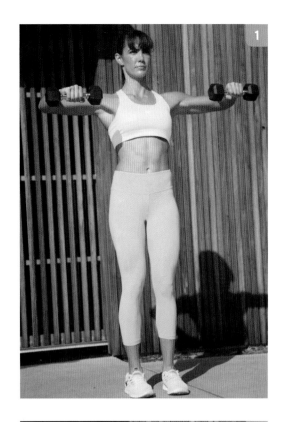

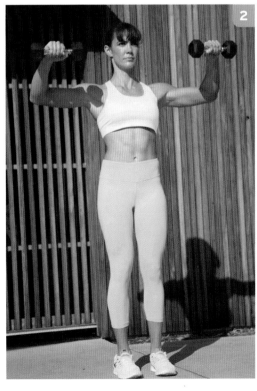

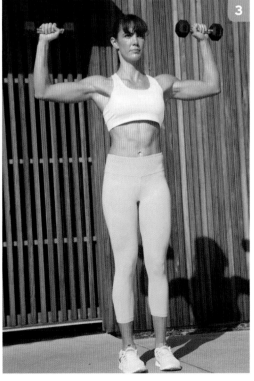

B4

Step up

Keeping one foot on the step or the bench, rotate the toe out slightly, keeping the weight in the heel at all times.

Step up using the working leg. The non-working leg should tap the bench quickly for 1 second, then lower down for 2 seconds.

Repeat 20 repetitions on each leg.

20, 4 sets, 2-0-1-0, 10 sec rest

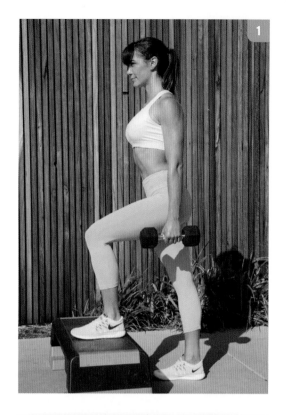

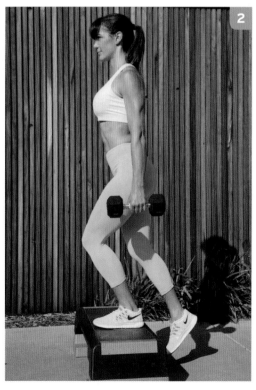

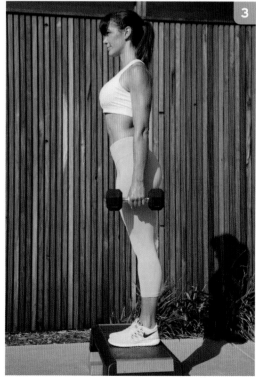

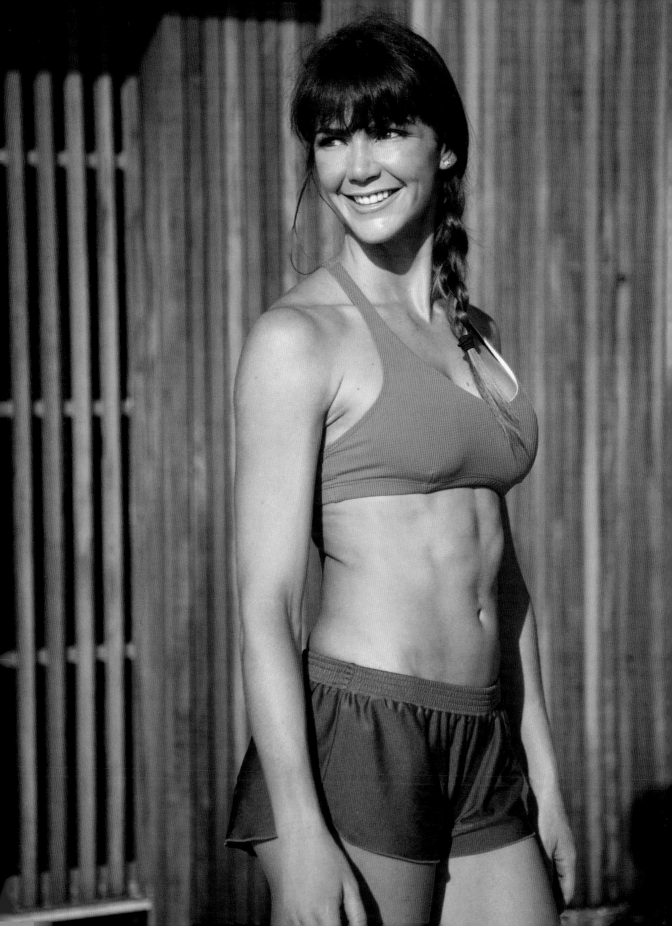

shredder shock work-out 1 (SSWO 1)

There are only three stations in this Shredder Shock Work-out. Complete all the As, then all the Bs, then all the Cs three times each in under 20 minutes or for time - that is, as fast as you can! This will get your heart rate up so you burn more calories and fat.

Sal's QUICK TIP . . . .

Ten seconds rest basically gives you the time to transition from one exercise to the next as fast as you can.

A1

100 skips

Jump rope!

If not using any equipment or you prefer not to use a rope, do a pretend skip.

100 reps, 3 sets, 10 sec rest

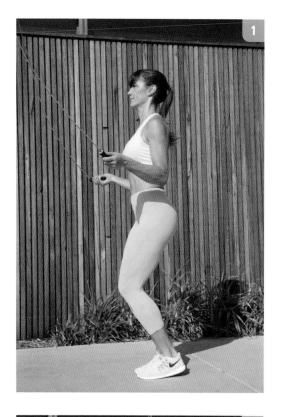

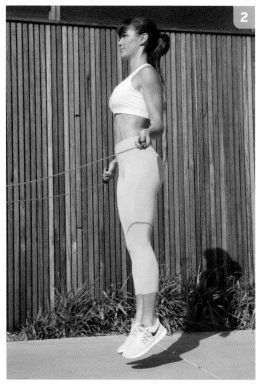

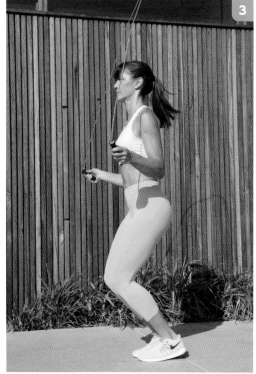

A2

Bench burpee

Keep the arms shoulder width apart on the bench.

Lower the body down fast and explode into a jump-up. Jump the feet out, and then lower the body down to repeat the movement.

15, 3 sets, 10 sec rest

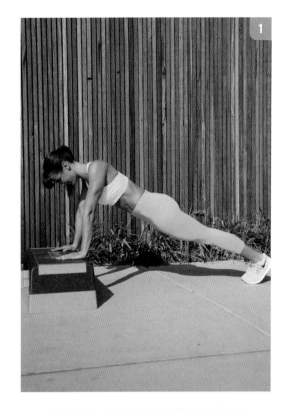

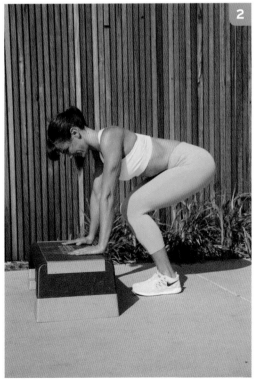

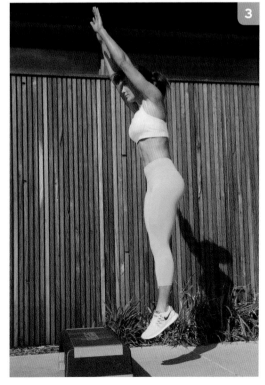

Box or step-jumps jump

Come into a semi squat, taking the weight into the heels then explode up, landing the feet onto the bench or box.

Step back down to the ground and repeat for 20 repetitions as fast as you can.

20, 3 sets, 10 sec rest

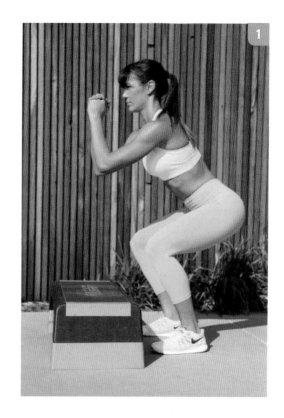

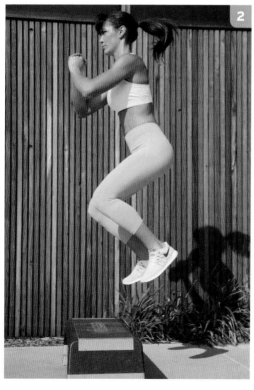

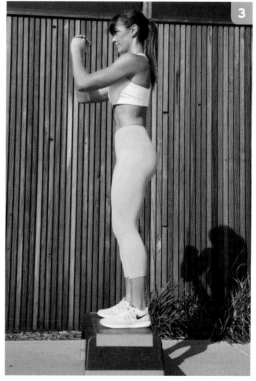

B1

Lunge jumps (front foot elevated, alternating)

Elevate the front foot onto a step or a bench.

Lower the body weight into the front heel and drive (or explode) through the top leg, quickly alternating with the other leg.

Repeat 20 times in total.

20, 3 sets, 10 secs rest

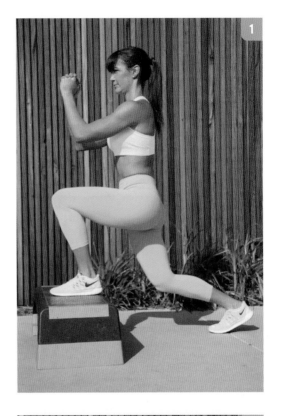

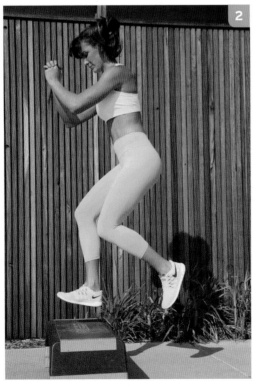

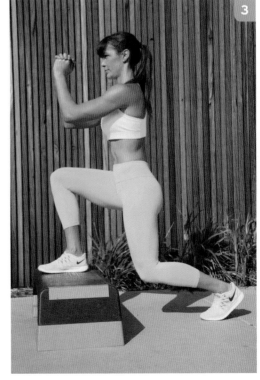

healthy body: balance your hormones and shred fat for life

Modified bench burpee box-jump with push-up

Keep the arms shoulder width apart on bench.

Lower the body down slowly with the target point being the chest to the bench, then explode into a jump-up.

Jump the feet onto the step, step down, then jump the feet back. Get back into your original position and repeat the movement.

10, 3 sets, 10 sec rest

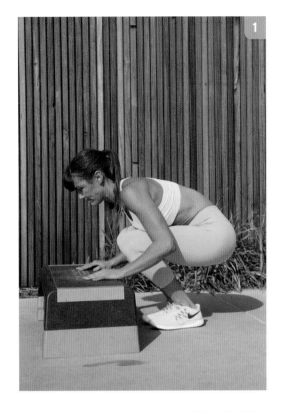

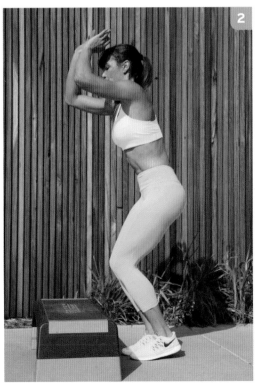

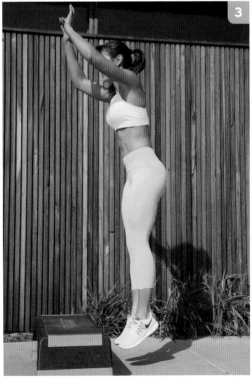

B3

Side step-overs

Keep one leg on the step at all times.

Explode up, using the leg on top of the step to quickly switching the legs so the other leg replaces the original leg on the step.

20, 3 sets, 10 sec rest

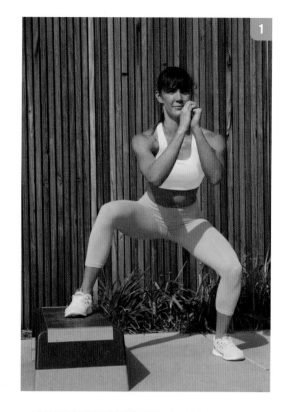

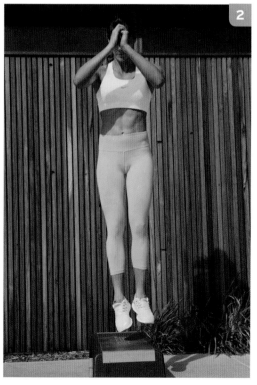

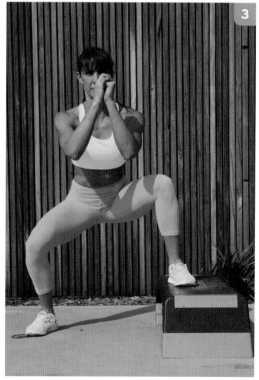

healthy body: balance your hormones and shred fat for life

C1

Squat jumps

Stand with the feet wide, toes turned out slightly and weight into the heels.

Squat down as far as you can keeping the chest upright and drive through the heels, exploding up into a jump.

15, 3 sets, 10 sec rest

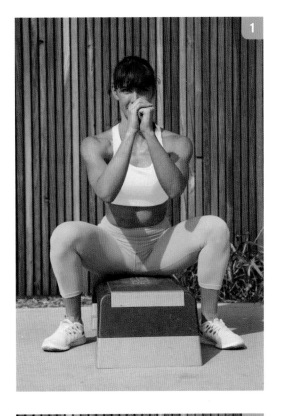

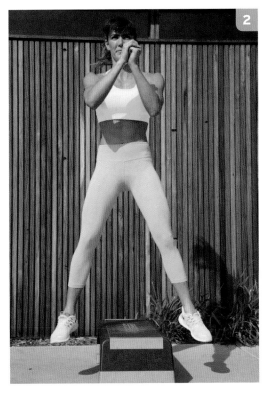

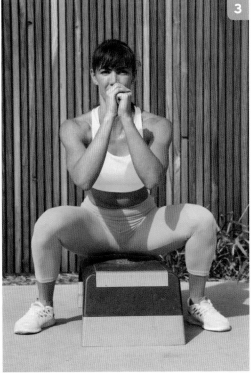

C2

Split jump squats on bench

Take one leg (back leg) onto the step. On the front leg or the working leg, lunge down first, then explode up as high as you can. Complete 10 repetitions as fast as you can keeping the hips in line and your weight through the heel. Switch legs and repeat.

10 each leg, 3 sets, 10 sec rest

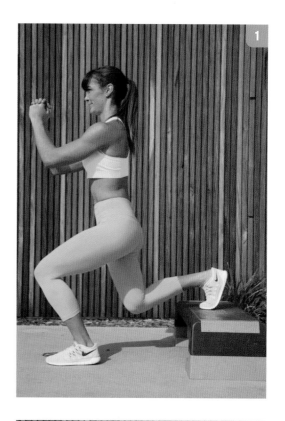

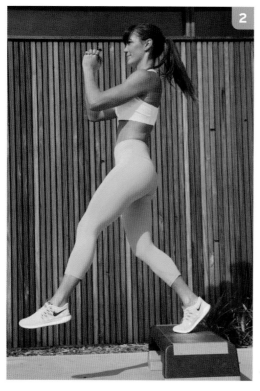

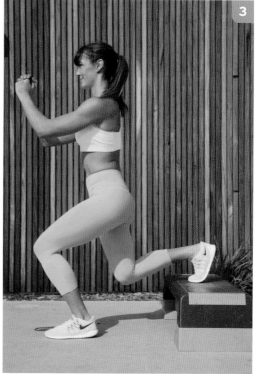

healthy body: balance your hormones and shred fat for life

Jump step

Keep one leg on top of the step and drive up through the heel. Keep the focus on the top leg, driving up through the heel, lifting the knee of the non-working leg. Repeat on the opposite leg. Complete 15 repetitions on each leg.

15 each leg, 3 sets, 10 sec rest each leg

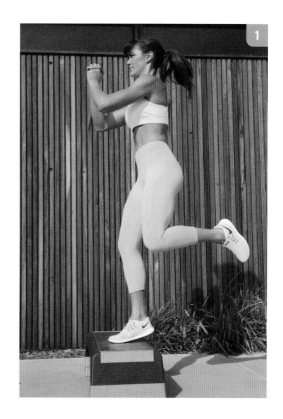

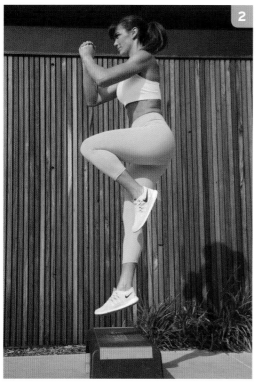

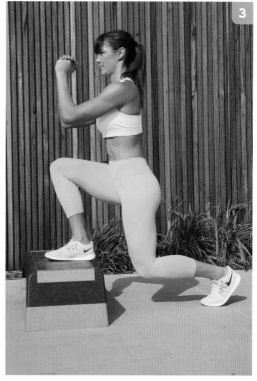

days 2 & 5

hamstrings glutes and shoulders + SSWO 2

First complete the four-station A circuits, four times through. Then move through the four-station B circuits, four times through.

Follow this up with SSWO 2, if desired. Complete all the As in the three-station circuit, then all the Bs, then all the Cs in under 20 minutes or for time – that is, as fast as you can!

A1

Shoulder press neutral

Start with the dumbbells on the shoulder line and press up for 1 second.

Keep the movement in an arch-like motion bringing the dumbbells together at the top of the range and lowering down to the starting position.

12, 4 sets, 4-0-1-0, 10 sec rest

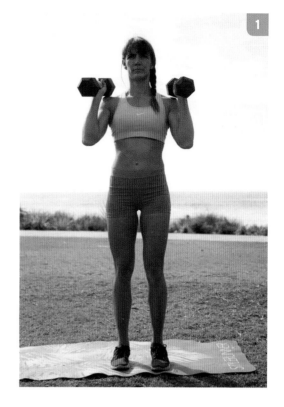

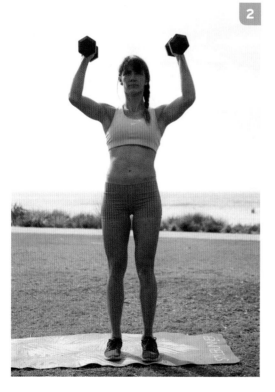

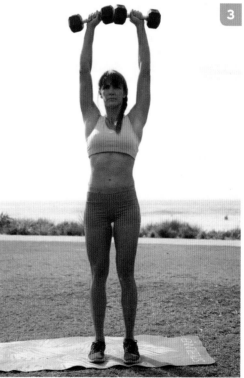

A2

Fitball curl feet

Lying face up, place both heels onto the fitball and bridge the hips up so that the body is in one straight line.

Contract the glutes and using the heel to dig, roll the ball into the glutes keeping a firm contraction on the muscles.

15, 4 sets, 3-0-1-0, 10 sec rest

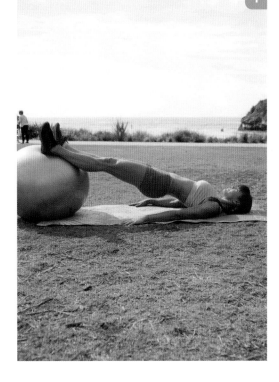

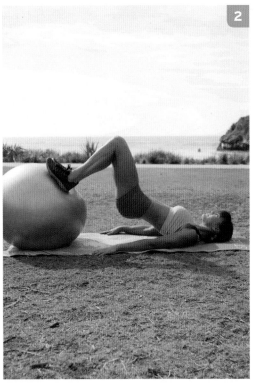

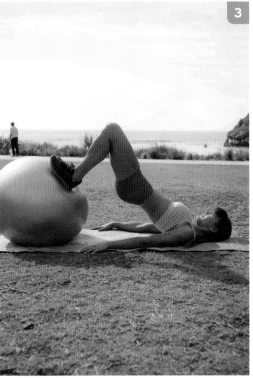

Behind-the-neck press with dumbbells

Hold dumbbells at the shoulder line and squeeze the shoulder blades together in preparation for the lift.

Draw the shoulders away from the ears and press the dumbbells up for 1 second in a vertical line, focussing on the back of the shoulder or the rear deltoid.

Lower down for 4 seconds to the original starting point.

15, 4 sets, 3-0-1-0, 10 sec rest

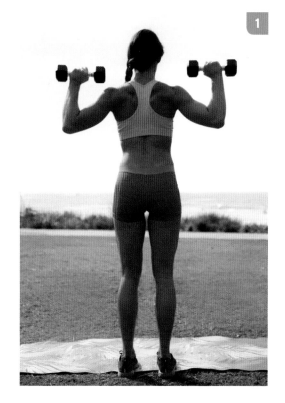

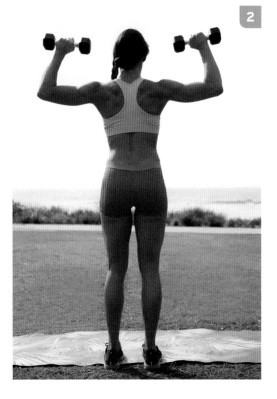

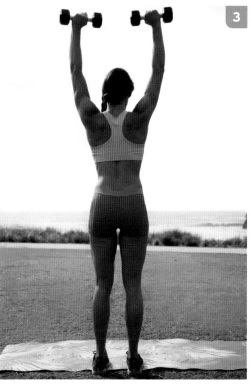

A4

Reverse hyper fitball

Lie prone or face down with your hips over the fitball like you are going into a lower-back stretch.

Bring your heels together into a v-shape and bring the legs up for 1 second, squeezing the glutes the entire time.

Lift the legs up until the body is in one straight line. Then lower down again for 3 seconds to the original position.

20, 4 sets, 3-0-1-0, 10 sec rest

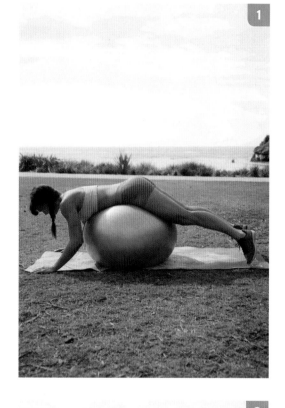

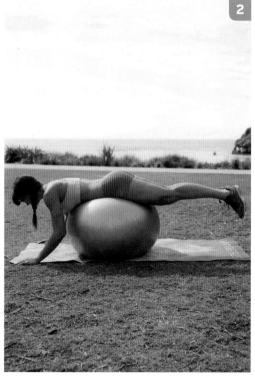

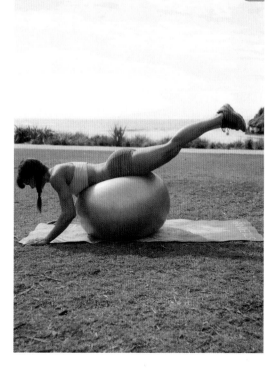

B1

Bent-over lateral raises on the fitball

Sit on the fitball and draw the navel into the spine. Tip from the hip, making sure that you are loading through the glutes and the hamstrings.

Keeping a slight bend at the elbow, bring the dumbbells just to the shoulder line, squeezing the back of the shoulders at all times.

Lower down for 4 sets, ensuring that you keep engaging the rear deltoid or the back of the shoulder.

12, 4 sets, 4-0-1-0, 10 sec rest

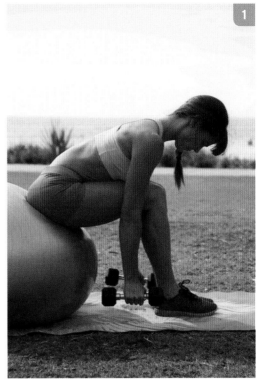

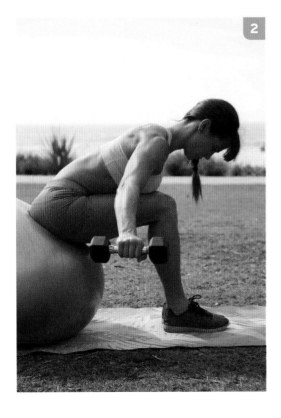

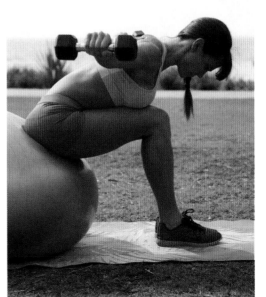

Hip thrusts with plate

Keep the plate in front of the body, ensuring the shoulder blades are pulled together the whole time.

Tip from the hip for 2 seconds, loading through the heels.

Keep focussing on the tip from the hip and drive through the heel for 1 second standing upright. Squeeze the glutes as you stand up to vertical.

15, 4 sets, 2-0-1-0, 10 sec rest

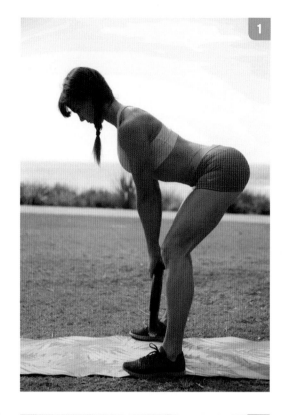

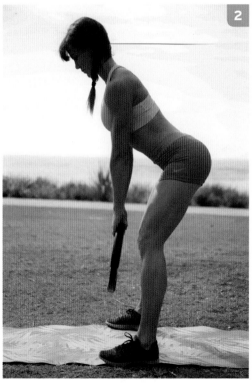

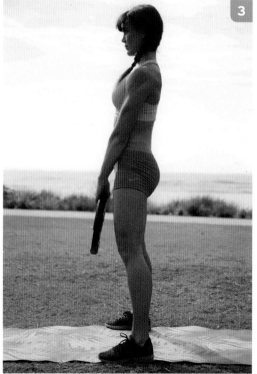

Front raise with dumbbell

Stand with your feet shoulder width apart, making sure your weight is through the heels and your tummy pulled in tight.

Keep the arms just outside the shoulder line.

Raise the arms just to your shoulder line, contracting the front of the shoulder for 1 second, then lower back down for 2 seconds.

20, 4 sets, 2-0-1-0, 10 sec rest

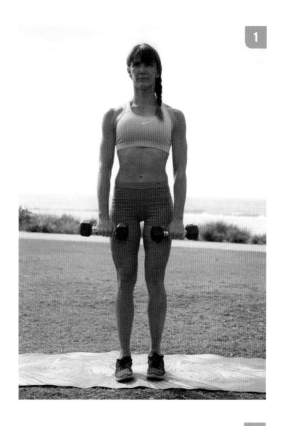

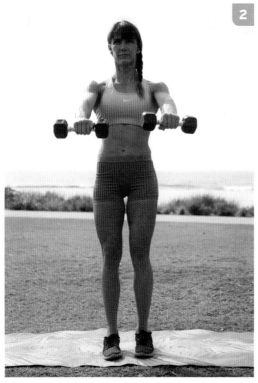

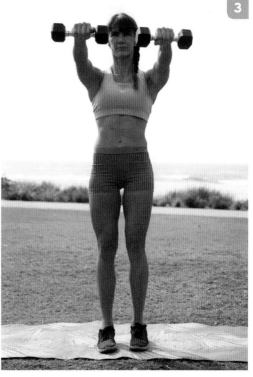

B4

Hip bridge on fitball

Lying face up, bring both feet onto the fitball.

Keep the ball in close to the body, weight into the heels. Drive up through the heels into a bridge for 1 second, then lower down for 2 seconds.

20, 4 sets, 2-0-1-0, 10 sec rest

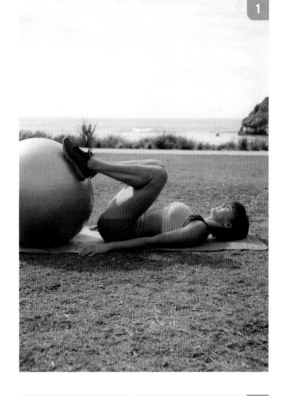

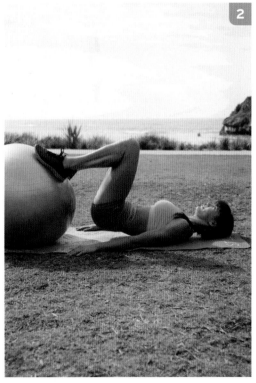

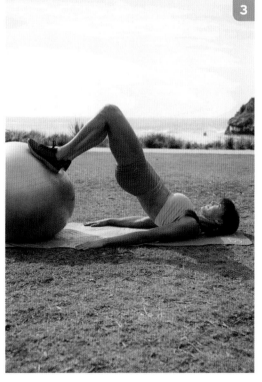

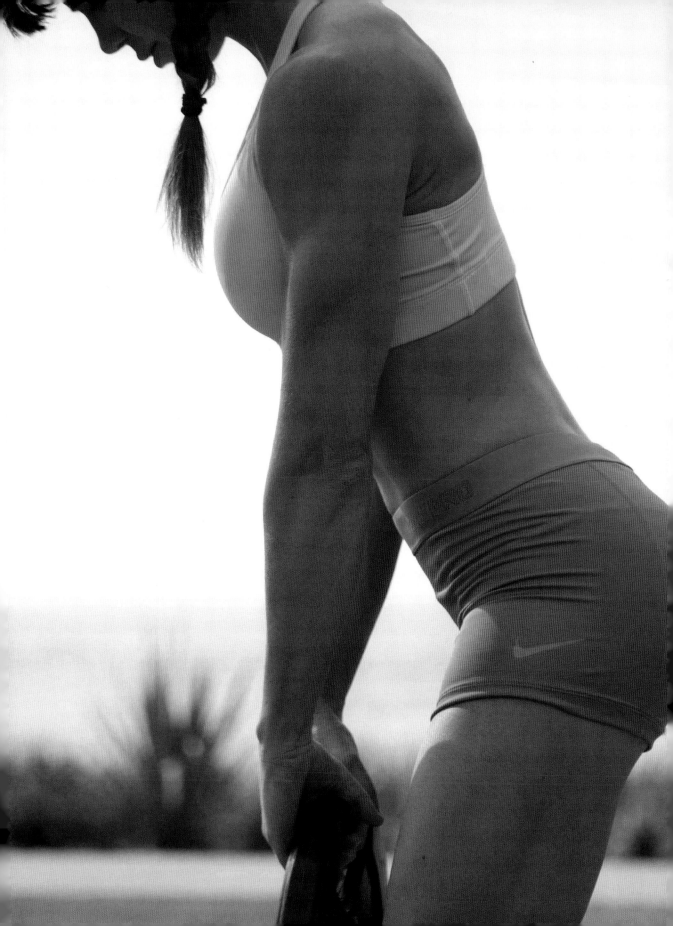

shredder shock work-out 2 (SSWO 2)

There are only three stations in this Shredder Shock Work-out. Complete all the As, then all the Bs, then all the Cs three times each in under 20 minutes or for time - that is, as fast as you can! This will get your heart rate up so you burn more calories and fat.

Sal's QUICK TIP

Ten seconds rest basically gives you the time to transition from one exercise to the next as fast as you can.

A1

Alternating step-ups

Start with one leg on the bench.

Jump high, leading with the top leg. Quickly switch or alternate legs as fast as you can for 20 repetitions (10 on each leg).

10 on each leg, 3 sets, 10 sec rest

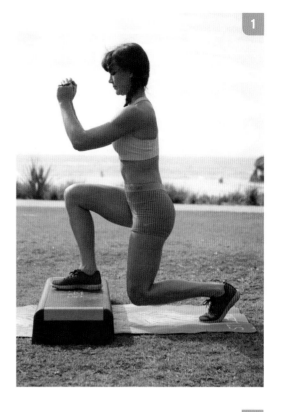

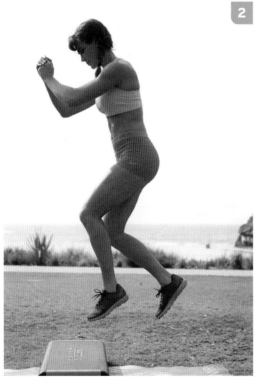

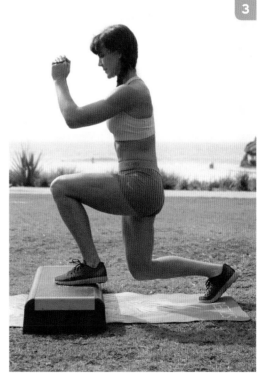

Mountain climbing

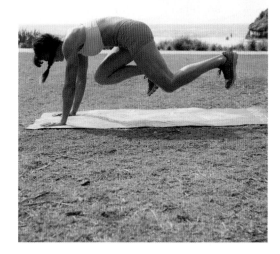

Get into a push-up or plank position, keeping the body in one straight line.

Alternate the knees into the chest as fast as you can, keeping the backside down and the tummy pulled in tight.

Repeat 20 times as fast as you can (10 on each leg).

10 on each leg, 3 sets, 10 sec rest

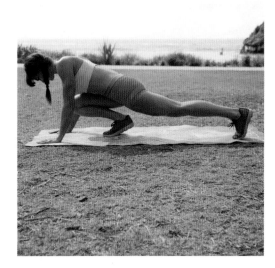

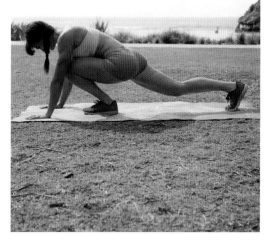

A3

Leaps

Start in a squat or crouched position.

From the ground, leap or jump as high as you can, taking the arms into the air at full extension. Repeat 20 times as fast as you can.

20, 3 sets, 10 sec rest

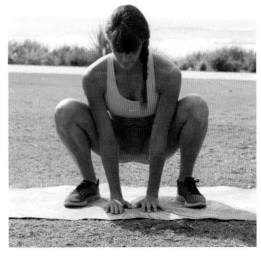

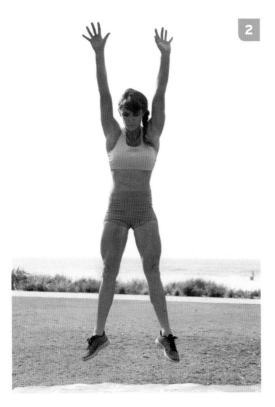

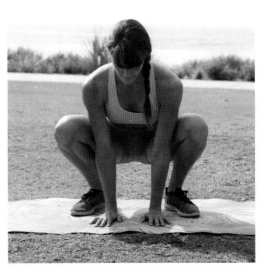

Lunge jumps

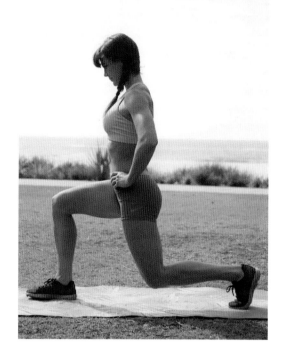

Stand in a split stance one foot forward, one foot back.

Lunge down through the back foot so that both legs are at 90 degrees. Quickly switch leg positions and lunge down into the original position.

Repeat 20 times in total (10 lunges on each leg).

10 on each leg, 3 sets, 10 sec rest

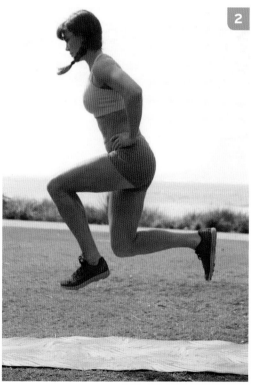

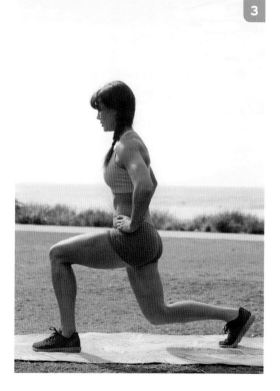

Modified burpee with chest push-up

Using a bench, take the arms wider than shoulder width into a push-up position.

Lower down, controlled. Then from that pushup position, drive up into a jump as high as you can. Jump the legs back to the original position and repeat 10 times in total.

10, 3 sets, 10 sec rest

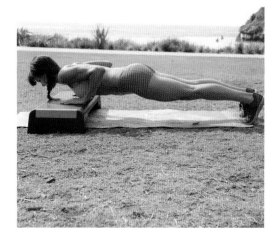

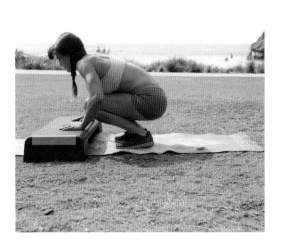

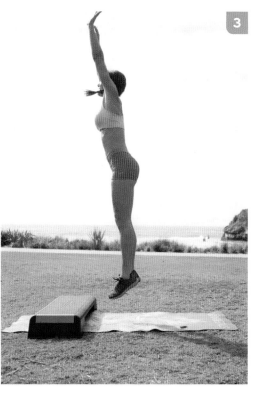

Alternating forward lunges

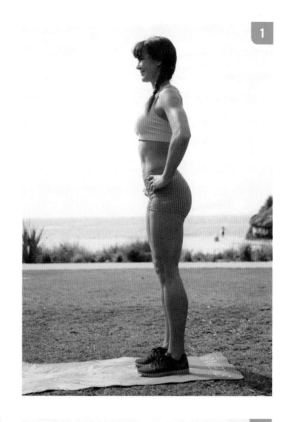

Start in the lunge position, one foot forward, one foot back.

Keep the focus through the front foot and take the toe out at a slight angle.

Lunge into the front leg then drive back through the heel, taking it into the front foot. Alternate legs until you reach 20 repetitions total (10 on each leg).

10 on each leg, 3 sets, 10 sec rest

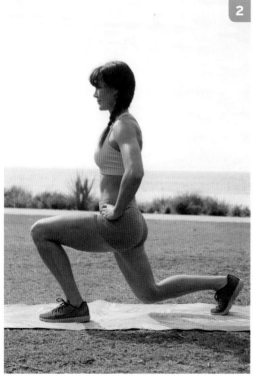

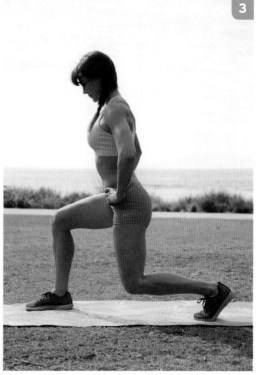

C1

Reverse lunge on bench

The front leg will be the working leg. Place the back leg (the non-working leg) on top of the step. Lower the back leg down into a lunge position, then quickly drive up through the heel on the front leg, squeezing the glutes to the starting position.

Ensure the weight is in the heel the entire time and the chest remains high, shoulders back and down. Perform 10 repetitions on each leg.

10 on each leg, 3 sets, 10 sec rest

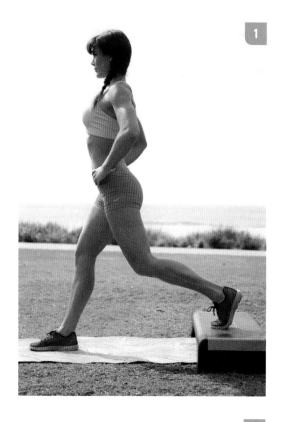

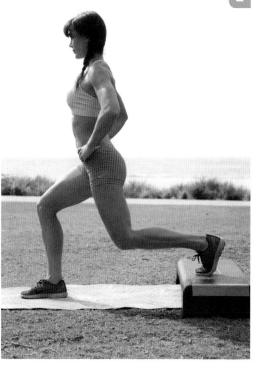

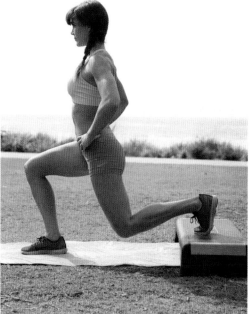

Side lunge jumps

Using a bench, keep one leg on top of the bench or step.

Lunge out to the side. Drive through the top leg quickly, switching the legs so that the leg comes into the side lunge once again. Perform 10 repetitions on each leg.

10 on each leg, 3 sets, 10 sec rest

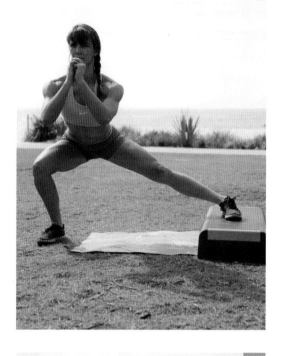

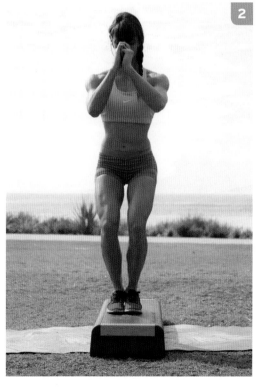

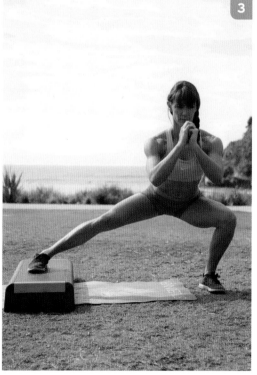

C3

High knees

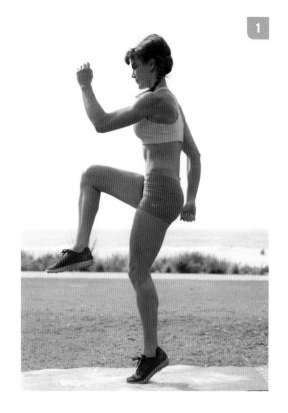

Keeping the chest proud, shoulders back, tummy in tight, lift the knees as high and as fast as you can. Make sure the body stays in a vertical line the entire time.

Repeat 20 times (10 on each leg). Complete in under 20 mins or for time (ie as fast as you can).

10 on each leg, 3 sets, 10 sec rest

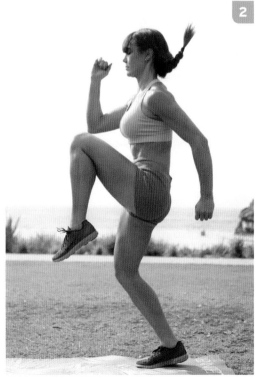

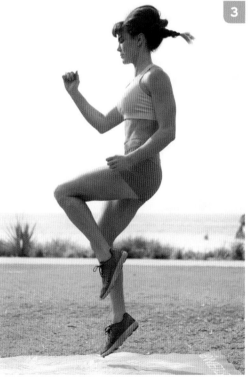

day 3

arms and abs

+ SSWO 3

First complete the four-station A circuits, four times through. Then move through the four-station B circuits, four times through.

Follow this up with SSWO 3, if desired. This is one circuit only to be done in 8-10 rounds through in under 20 minutes or for time - that is, as fast as you can!

A1

Tricep push-up with bench

Bring hands onto the bench, no wider than shoulder width apart.

Keeping the body in one straight line, lower down for 3 seconds and up for 1 second.

Shoulders should remain down and back, aiming the chest between the hands.

12, 4 sets, 3-0-1-0, 10 sec rest

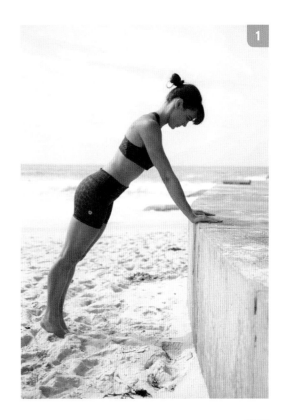

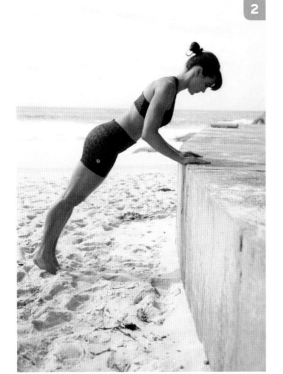

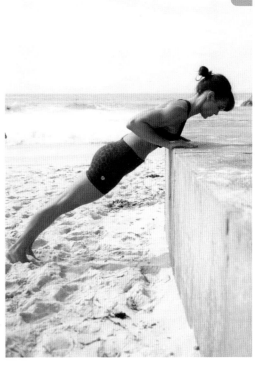

Tricep dip with bench

Keeping your back close to the bench and body vertical, lower the body down for 3 seconds and up for 1. Keep the elbows in close together and imagine that there is something between the elbows like a bowling ball.

(There is always the temptation for the back to come away from the bench – always make sure you keep the body close to the bench at all times.)

15, 4 sets, 3-0-1-0, 10 sec rest

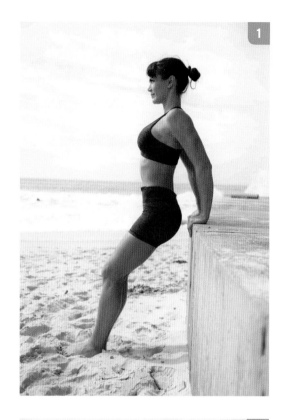

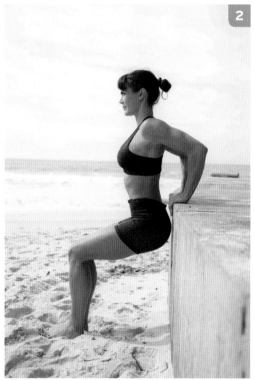

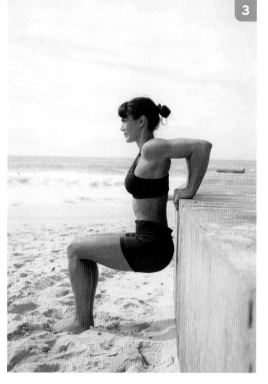

French press with dumbbell

Hold the weighted part of the dumbbell and carefully place over the head.

Squeeze the elbows tightly together, lowering the weight down for 3 seconds and up for 1 second.

Make sure the elbow does not move. Contract the triceps as you extend the arm.

20, 4 sets, 3-0-1-0, 10 sec rest

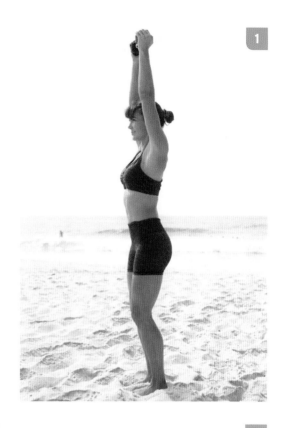

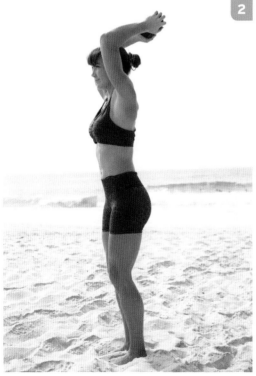

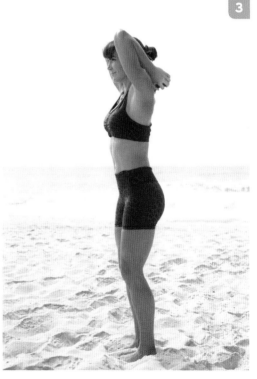

Tricep kick-back bilateral (both arms)

Tip from the hip and load through the glutes and hamstrings.

Making sure the load is through the heels, bring the arms up to a 90-degree angle. Extend the elbows until the arms are completely straight.

Contract the triceps and the back of the arms in this position.

20, 4 sets, 2-0-1-0, 10 sec rest

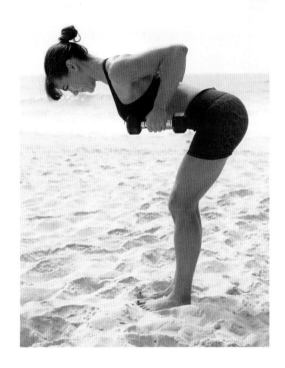

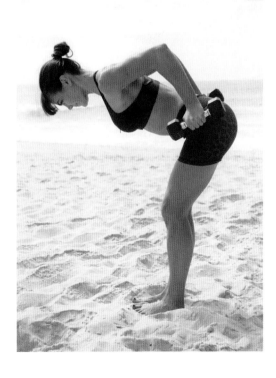

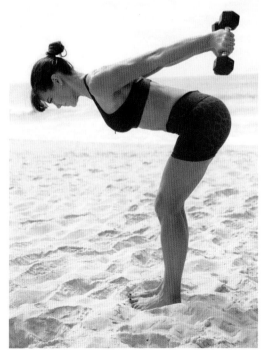

Neutral grip dumbbell curl

Standing with your feet wider than shoulder width apart, soften the knees and keep the tummy in tight. Draw the shoulder down and back.

Keeping the weights in a neutral position, bring the dumbbells up to the shoulders for 1 second and down for 3 seconds.

15, 4 sets, 3-0-1-0, 10 sec rest

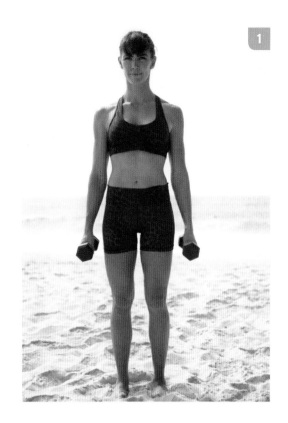

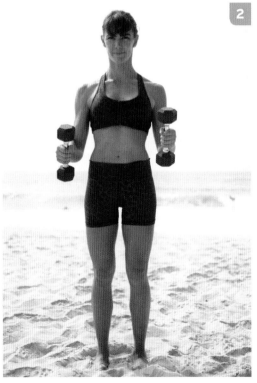

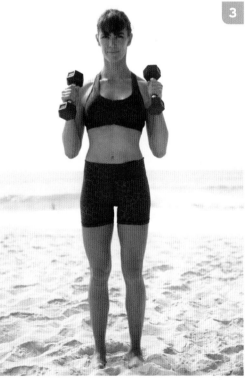

Fitball curl

Sit on the fitball.

Contract the abdominals before you get into the crunch position.

Walk the feet forward so that you position the fitball into the lower back.

From that position, use the abdominals to lift yourself up to a 45-degree angle and contract the abdominals. Then lower the ball back down for 4 seconds.

15, 4 sets, 4-0-1-0, 10 sec rest

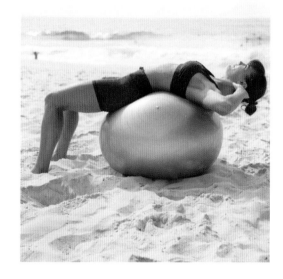

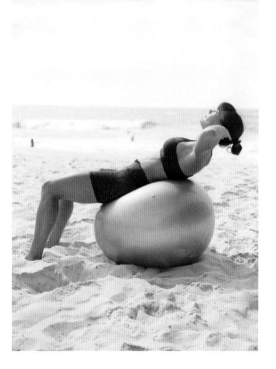

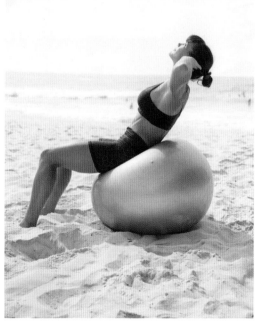

B3

Zottman curl
with dumbbell

Stand with your feet hip distance apart.

Bend slightly at the knee joint, shoulders down and back.

Start with the dumbbells in a neutral position and as you lift the weight, rotate the weights to a supinated position up to the shoulder line.

Lower down the same way for 2 seconds back to your original position.

20, 4 sets, 2-0-1-0, 10 sec rest

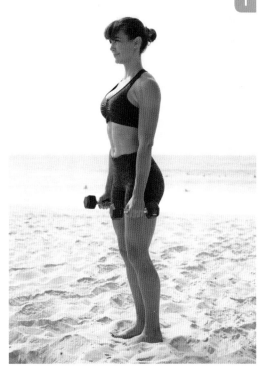

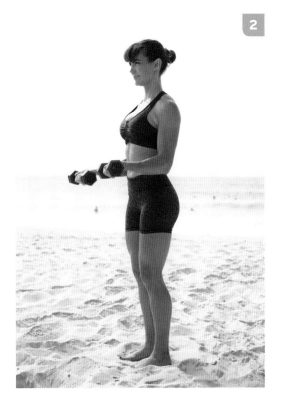

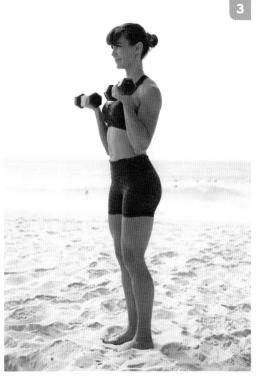

B4

Reverse curl
(legs at 90 degrees)

Lying down on your back, bring the knees up to 90 degrees.

Lower one leg down until the heel is just off the ground. Ensure the lower back remains flat at all times. Repeat alternating legs.

Complete 20 repetitions total (ie 10 on each leg).

20, 4 sets, 3-0-1-0, 10 sec rest

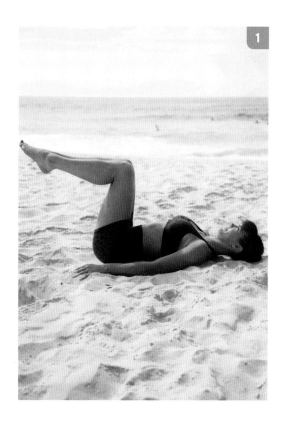

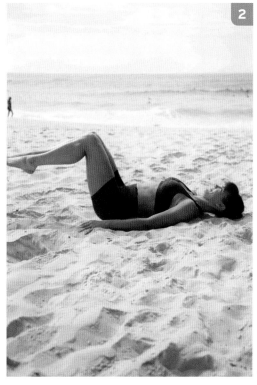

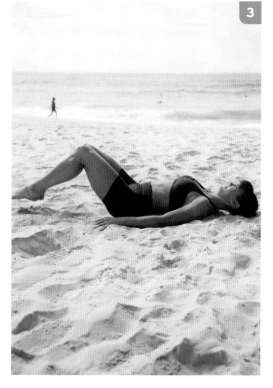

healthy body: balance your hormones and shred fat for life

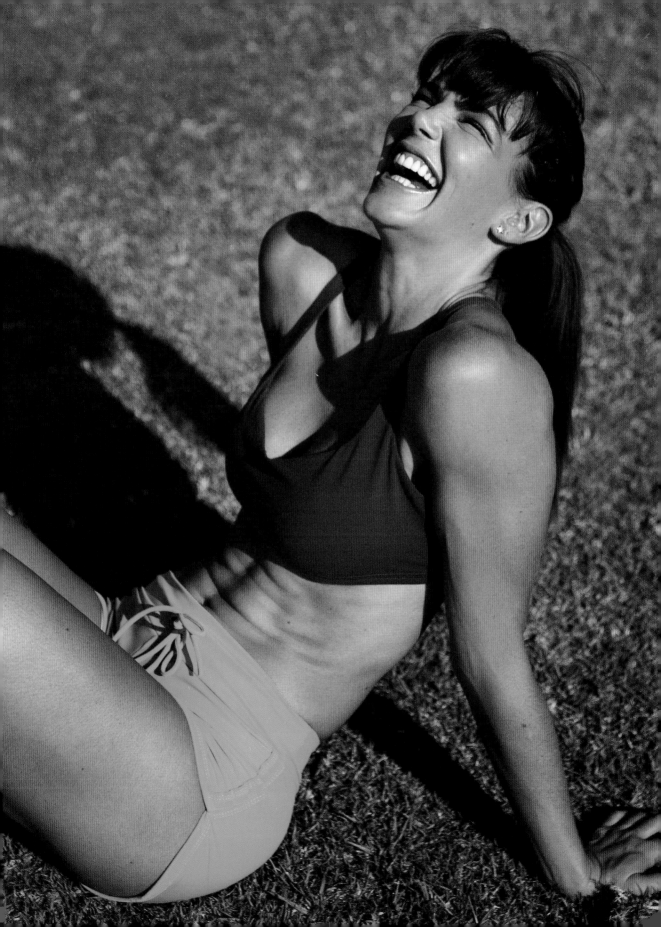

shredder shock work-out 3 (SSWO 3)

This is one circuit only to be done in 8-10 rounds through.

Sal's QUICK TIP . . . .

You will perform both A1 and A2 for a 20-second effort, then you will lunge walk back to your starting position (this is your A3 exercise).

A1

Incline run (stair or hill)

Ensure posture is upright and shoulders are down and back.

Keeping the chest proud, run. Make sure you are striking the middle of the foot either on the hill or stair. Keep the knees lifted high and focus on contracting the abdominals and glutes as you run.

20 seconds, 8-10 sets, 10 sec rest

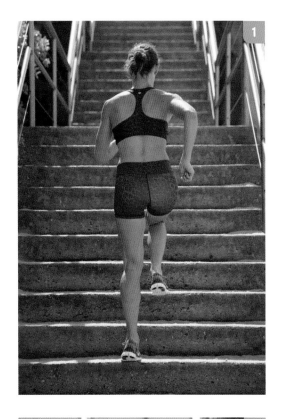

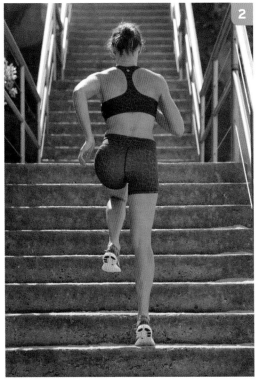

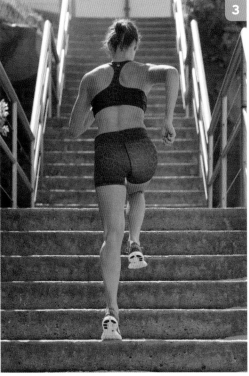

A2

Flat run

Ensure posture is upright and shoulders are down and back.

Keeping the chest proud, run. Make sure you are striking the middle of the foot directly on the (flat) ground. Keep the knees lifted high and focus on contracting the abdominals and glutes as you run.

20 seconds, 8-10 sets, 10 sec rest

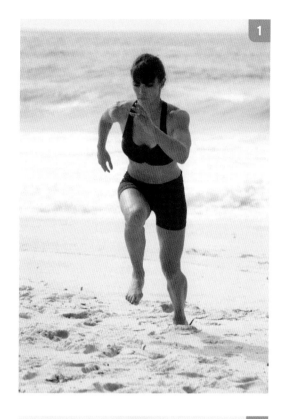

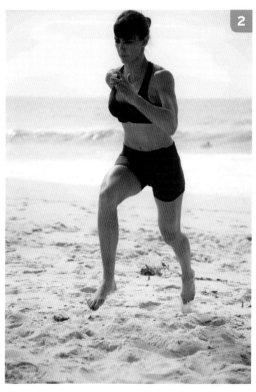

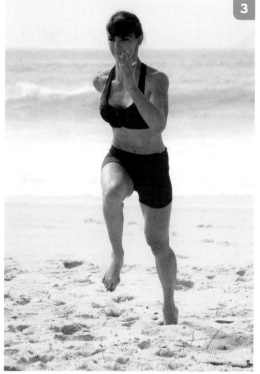

A3

Walking lunge using body weight

Placing one slightly turned-out foot in front of the other, lower or lunge down into the front heel for 2 seconds then drive up for 1, keeping the weight in the heel.

Repeat the lunge walking, alternating for the full length of the 20-second effort run in A2

Return to starting position, 8-10 sets, 10 sec rest

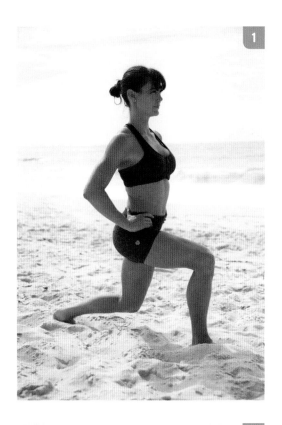

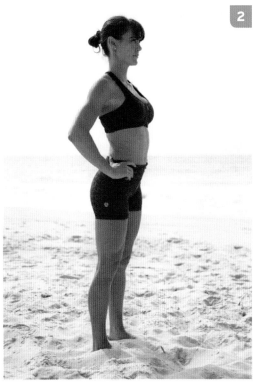

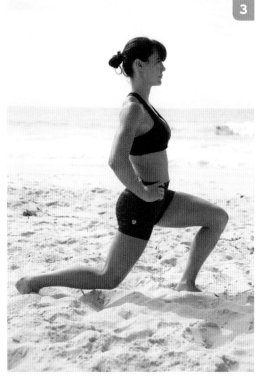

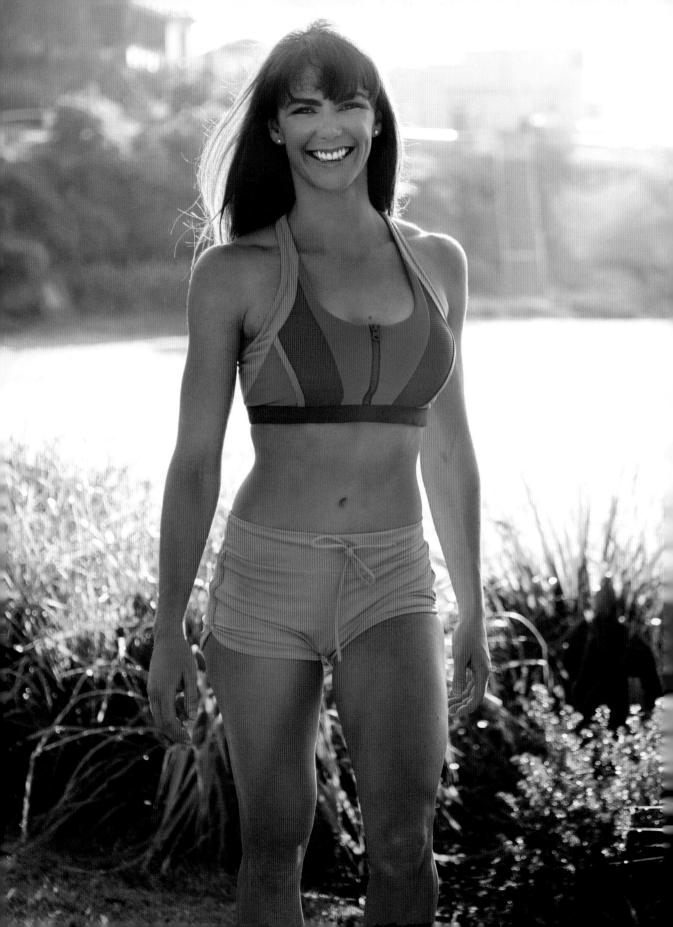

chapter **3**

stay lean
with the
right
nutrition

**My food philosophy is all about
lifestyle changes, not diets.**

Nutrition is, without a doubt, 80% of the battle. Get that right and you are cruising on the super fat-burning highway. By focussing on what you eat and how you supplement your nutritional needs, you can take control of your body and your health.

PROTEIN IS OF UTMOST IMPORTANCE

Protein is made up of branch chain amino acids that are vital for healthy body function. They can also help accelerate fat loss as, put simply, protein doesn't stimulate insulin.

It is therefore absolutely critical that you hit your protein targets daily (see the meal plans below for extra guidance). You should be consuming:

- approximately 100-120g (3.5-4.25oz) of protein a day for the average female
- approximately 240-260g (8.5-9oz) for the average male.

In raw weight, this equates to:

- approximately 500-600g (1.1-1.3lb) per day for the average female, depending on the quality of the protein.
- approximately 800-900g (1.75-2lb) per day for the average male, depending on the quality of the protein.

As a general guide, there is approximately 22-30g (0.75-1oz) of protein in every 100g (3.5oz) of raw animal meat and in one whole egg, there is approximately 6g (0.2oz).

> ### *Sal's* QUICK TIP
>
> Our ancestors ate a lot of meat, plant-based carbs, nuts and seeds and I don't know about you, but I don't recall any cavemen - or women! - with man boobs or muffin tops.

I am not a massive fan of weighing food. My food philosophy is all about *lifestyle changes, not diets*. In fact, I want you to get comfortable measuring the correct portions simply by sight, so I have included an easy visual guide below.

Protein sight scale

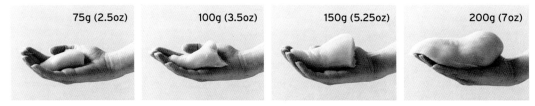

| 75g (2.5oz) | 100g (3.5oz) | 150g (5.25oz) | 200g (7oz) |

In addition to hitting your protein target in at least 4-5 meals throughout the day, make consuming leafy green vegetables a priority for your daily fibre intake, along with grain-less fibre sources such as chia seeds or slippery elm.

Sal's QUICK TIP . . . .

If you are struggling to hit your protein targets, a good quality, easily digestible whey protein powder can help. Use on its own as a snack throughout the day (eg meals 2 or 4) or as a supplement in cooking (see also: Snacks).

CHOOSE YOUR CARBS AND FATS WISELY

Eat right - and at the right time - to improve your hormone health. Following is some general advice to guide you on your way that will help you regardless of where you are storing fat.

- Plant-based carbohydrates and good fats in the morning can increase *dopamine* levels - the hormone responsible for attention and productivity.
- Starchy carbs like sweet potato in the evening can help release *serotonin* - the feel-good hormone that helps you to relax at night and sleep better as well as lower cortisol levels.
- Good fats (such as unsaturated fats from fish, seeds, nuts, leafy vegetables, some oils and avocadoes) can actually help you burn fat.

Getting your dopamine and serotonin levels right can help control your moods as well as balance other hormones such as cortisol. Even better, the more we eat foods that fuel and balance hormonal activity, the better our body's ability to burn fat.

Sal's QUICK TIP . . . .

Of course, if you suspect you may have some hormonal imbalances, it is advisable to get your blood work done with a GP.

Note that if you have starchy foods (or when you reintroduce them back into the diet regularly, for example once you have reached your target body fat), the two optimal times to eat them are:

- within 30 minutes of training, as it will replenish the body's glycogen stores
- at your evening meal, as it well help relax the body by releasing serotonin and improving sleep.

TOO MUCH FRUCTOSE CAN HINDER YOUR PROGRESS

Fructose is a sugar that is found in large quantities in processed foods in the form of corn syrup, but it is also present in fruit. Unfortunately, the body responds to fructose, especially in large quantities, by turning it straight into fat.

It also alters liver function and, if you eat large quantities regularly, it will upset the liver and make it harder to process glucose (energy from carbs) - meaning you'll get even fatter in the long run.

Sals QUICK TIP . . . .

Keep fructose to a bare minimum. Studies show the best time to eat fructose is after exertion or training. The body processes it more efficiently at this time, helping replenish energy stores quickly.

GLUTEN IS NOT YOUR FRIEND

Have you ever eaten a bowl of pasta or a sandwich and wondered why you really bloated out? Maybe you feel like this all the time? It is possible you feel like this because of the food you ingest, in particular, gluten.

Gluten is found in many staple foods in the western diet. It is a protein composite present in wheat and other grains. Gluten is big in the bread world - it gives elasticity to dough, helps it to rise and stay in shape. It's like the glue that sticks wheat together, literally. Unfortunately, it doesn't help us stay in shape. In fact, quite the opposite.

While you may not be a coeliac (someone who suffers from a severe intolerance to gluten) you could still be gluten sensitive. In fact, if you ask me, most people are. Gluten is hard for our bodies to digest, makes us tired, bloats the belly and, most importantly, adds extra weight and puffiness to our physique. It can also cause illness and sometimes, it can even influence your mental health.

THE WORD ON FATS

Fat free really means full of sugar and artificial fluff. It's a trap that a lot of people fall into - they think they are saving on calories but wonder why they can't shift the weight for good.

Basically, when you fill yourself up with sugar and carbs (and this includes fruit), you spike your insulin levels. Studies have shown that insulin is the main culprit of fat production, particularly around that pesky mid-section, so to counteract this you need to control the carbs, crush the sugar, ignore the calories and welcome in the good fats.

Sal's QUICK TIP ....

Forget fat free. Good fats can actually help you lose weight.

This is why you will notice that in my recipes I use a variety of different cooking oils. I generally recommend rotating different oils or browning agents as you would protein sources, providing a range of health benefits as well as flavours in the meals.

- Organic butter is one of the best - and one of my favourite - methods of browning food and adding flavour, as it contains iodine. This is great for stimulating the thyroid, which in turn helps boost your metabolism.
- Grapeseed oil is known for its high smoke point and although it does not have the health benefits of other oils, it is good for frying things that require a high heat.
- Coconut oil has many health benefits, and is known for its ability to be heated and not turn into an unhealthy trans fat. (Trans fats are the bad form of cholesterol that decrease your good cholesterol, the high-density lipoprotein.)
- Olive oils are best used cold (not heated) as they are known for their antioxidant properties when used in this way.
- Flaxseed oil is another great oil of choice, which again, when not overheated, is very high in good fats.

As always, variety and moderation is key.

ALCOHOL

Alcohol is a toxin. As such, your body will always process it through your liver and kidneys first - the two vital organs that are also the main drivers of processing fat. So if your body is busy burning up alcohol, it is not shredding fat like it is supposed to.

Alcohol is also classified as empty calories - food that contains energy, but has little or no nutritional value. It is very easy to drink too much (this includes fruit juices and soft drinks too), which means you can quickly end up drinking more calories than you are burning off. The body then has no other option but to store that extra energy as fat.

If you must have a drink, I suggest clear spirits (they are lower in calories than beer and sugary ciders). Try vodka or gin mixed with freshly squeezed lime or lemon mixed with mineral or soda water for fewer calories or with diet soft drinks. Avoid mixing your drinks with fruit juices or soft drinks.

Sal's QUICK TIP

Avoid cheaper vodkas as they are made from wheat, which contains gluten. The more expensive brands are generally made from potatoes and are therefore often better for overall digestion.

Dry red and white wine has little residual sugar and, in moderation, red wine has some benefits. Avoid champagne and sweet wines, including dessert wines.

The old tips to only half fill your glass and alternate each alcoholic drink with water are still sound messages. After all, it is all about balance, but keep in mind that your results will be more rapid if you remain alcohol-free.

Sal's QUICK TIP

My suggestion? Whether it is gluten or alcohol or anything else, if in doubt, leave it out. Especially if you want to fight the flab. You will feel so much better. Trust me.

SAMPLE MEAL PLANS

I have developed the following sample meal plans, one for the average female, and one for the average male. They should keep you on target throughout the day and get you started on the road to successful fat loss no matter where you are currently storing fat in your body.

The meal plans recommend eating three main meals and two snacks per day. If you are time poor and/or this is difficult for you, try focussing on eating three times a day instead. Just make sure you still hit your total daily protein target.

I suggest you follow the meal plan for six consecutive days out of seven. At the end of six days, you can include a load meal on a refuel day. Dinner is always my favourite time to reward myself.

This load meal on a refuel day can actually help your progress by feeding your muscles. It also tricks the body into using the extra energy from carbs for fuel, rather than storing them as body fat.

Sal's QUICK TIP

This process of carb control is extremely effective for fat loss and lean muscle development – it also gives you something to look forward to! You may find that once your body becomes a better fat-burning machine, you will wake up feeling leaner and tighter around your tummy. Just make sure that you keep it to one load meal on your refuel day to keep these results going.

It is still important to stick to your protein target on these days, but you can choose a calorie-dense meal such as a gluten-free pizza or pasta dish, fruit of any kind, honey or maple syrup, ice-cream (or other dairy), or dark chocolate. (See also our Treats and cheats recipes below.)

Basically, on these days, you can treat yourself to anything rich in calories and carbohydrates. This is your reward! Even better, shredders, it will actually help, not hinder your progress, so have a guilt-free treat and keep the body fuelled for fat loss, muscle development and toning.

Sal's QUICK TIP

Sugar cravings should lessen as you up your protein intake, but if you are battling the urge for something sweet, try adding cinnamon sticks or fresh lemon or lime to your drinking water. Research shows that this can help lower the insulin response to food and also stop the palate or taste buds wanting to reach for the chocolate and lollies. Peppermint tea after a meal can also help.

Sample FEMALE meal plan:
approximately 100-120g (3.5-4.25oz) protein

Total raw weight protein target per day: 500-600g (1.1-1.3lb)

Meal 1 (breakfast)

Start with 150g (5.25oz) raw measure of animal protein such as smoked salmon, turkey or beef (*see*: Sight scale).

Alternatively, two whole eggs contain approximately 12g (0.4oz) of protein.

Add a palm-size portion of good fats like nuts, avocado or haloumi, which is a great source of good fat and a fantastic breakfast option.

Mix things up by including some vegies like asparagus or parsley.

(*See also*: Breakfast recipes)

Meal 2 (snack)

Choose 75-100g (2.5-3.5oz) raw measure of protein (*see*: Sight scale) such as a tin of tuna or salmon.

Alternatively, try boiled eggs or the turkey cups if you are on the run. They are an excellent snack as you can eat them cold and they provide a decent hit of protein.

Mix and match with some good fats such as nuts, avocado, haloumi or feta and add in some carrot or celery sticks and cherry tomatoes.

(*See also*: Snack ideas)

Meal 3 (lunch)

Choose 150g (5.25oz) raw measure of protein (*see*: Sight scale).

Add some fibrous vegetables or salad.

Choose vinegar-based dressings or lemon or lime, to help reduce the glycaemic load on food.

(*See also*: Lunch and dinner recipes and ideas)

Meal 4 (snack)

Choose 75-100g (2.5-3.5oz) raw measure of protein (*see*: Sight scale) such as a tin of tuna or salmon.

Mix and match with some good fats such as nuts, avocado, haloumi or feta and add in some carrot or celery sticks and cherry tomatoes.

(*See also*: Snack ideas)

Meal 5 (dinner)

Choose 150g (5.25oz) raw measure of protein (see Sight scale).

Serve with vegies or salad drizzled with a good oil and vinegar if desired.

(*See also*: Lunch and dinner recipes)

Sample MALE meal plan:
approximately 240-260g (8.5-9oz) protein

Total raw weight protein target per day: 800-900 g (1.75-2lb)

Meal 1 (breakfast)

Start with 250g (8.75 oz) raw measure of animal protein such as smoked salmon, turkey or beef (*see*: Sight scale).

Alternatively, two whole eggs contain approximately 12g (0.4 oz) of protein.

Add a palm-size portion of good fats like nuts, avocado or haloumi, which is a great source of good fat and a fantastic breakfast option.

Mix things up by including some vegies like asparagus or parsley.

(*See also*: Breakfast recipes)

Meal 2 (snack)

Choose 100-150g (3.5-5.25oz) raw measure of protein (*see*: Sight scale) such as a tin of tuna or salmon. Alternatively, try boiled eggs.

Mix and match with some good fats such as nuts, avocado, haloumi or feta and add in some carrot or celery sticks and cherry tomatoes.

(*See also*: Snack ideas)

Meal 3 (lunch)

Choose 250g (8.75oz) raw measure of protein (*see*: Sight scale).

Add some fibrous vegetables or salad.

Choose vinegar-based dressings or lemon or lime, to help reduce the glycaemic load on food.

(*See also*: Lunch and dinner recipes and ideas)

Meal 4 (snack)

Choose 100-150g (3.5-5.25oz) raw measure of protein (*see*: Sight scale) such as a tin of tuna or salmon.

Mix and match with some good fats such as nuts, avocado, haloumi or feta and add in some carrot or celery sticks and cherry tomatoes.

(*See also*: Snack ideas)

Meal 5 (dinner)

Choose 250g (8.75oz) raw measure of protein (see Sight scale).

Serve with vegies or salad drizzled with a good oil and vinegar if desired.

(*See also*: Lunch and dinner recipes)

SUPPLEMENTS

In addition to the healthy meal plans, I suggest you combine your food intake with the following supplements to promote lean muscle development and shred fat. Taken at the right time of day, they can provide a multitude of benefits.

- A good digestion support (such as HCL) is the most important supplement. Without adequate amounts of good digestive acid, you will not absorb crucial vitamins and minerals.
- Fish oil can lower the production of insulin.
- Magnesium can promote relaxation and lower cortisol levels, which in turn can lower body fat.
- A good multivitamin with B vitamins, vitamin D and zinc promotes detoxification and therefore fat loss.
- Ensure adequate fibre by taking a supplement in soluble form (from your local supermarket or health food store).

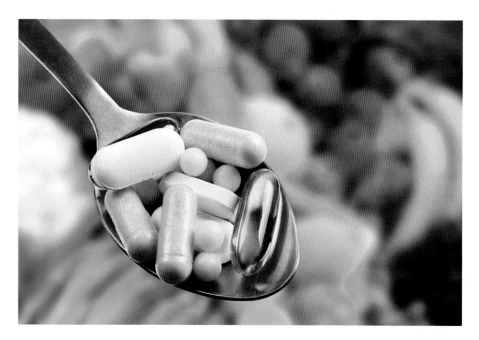

Taken at the right time of day, supplements can provide a multitude of benefits.

healthy body: balance your hormones and shred fat for life

I take my supplements throughout the day to ensure I have the energy to train - and recover - well. I also believe it gives me a better quality of life as I feel alert during the day and tired and relaxed at night. Try the following.

Pre-work-out

For morning work-outs, use an L-carnitine in capsule form up to 300-500 mg about 20-30 minutes before training. This increases potential fat loss during exercise as well as increasing attention and energy during training.

During your work-out

BCAA (branch chain amino acids) can improve recovery.

The amino acid L-leucine has been shown to burn visceral fat.

Amino acids (up to 3000 mg a day) can also promote liver detoxification, leading to greater fat loss.

With meals

I recommend eating half your meal and then taking the supplements suggested below at breakfast, lunch and dinner.

- EPA-dominant, pharmaceutical-grade omega-3 fish oil (600-1000 mg).
- A good multivitamin (300-600 mg).
- A good digestion support such as HCL (300-600 mg).

At dinner only, include magnesium. I suggest starting with a modest dose of 300-600 mg a day. However, in extremely magnesium-deficient people, I have found up to 4000 mg a day to be a safe and effective way to restore appropriate levels, while also helping mood and sleep disorders.

Before bed

I recommend taking a grainless, soluble fibre 30 minutes before bed with water. Choose two different types and rotate every seven days as after this time, it stops having the same effect on the body.

THINGS TO KEEP IN MIND

I have noticed a massive change in my physique and overall wellbeing over time. My main take-home points to help you on your health and wellness journey towards fat loss are as follows.

Keep going, shredders, you can do it!

- The use of *supplementation* specifically for fat loss ensures that you are actually absorbing the vitamins and minerals in your food and is highly recommended (see above).

- *Digestion and detoxification* are the two essentials for fat loss. Proper digestion ensures you are absorbing vital vitamins and minerals to help speed up the fat loss process and detoxification makes sure you are excreting nasty toxins that can also lead to stubborn fat gain. In fact, starting your day with a protein breakfast ensures your body begins detoxing from the get-go as the amino acids in the protein will start toxin elimination through the kidneys and liver.

- Think of your body like a car: it needs refuelling throughout the day to keep it in top gear and to *make sure your metabolism, or engine, is running at its optimum level.* (For this reason, and for long term fat loss, I don't recommend intermittent fasting.)

- Remember to *eat your protein first*, rotating your choice of protein regularly.

- For both men and women, it is *all-you-can-eat vegies and salads.* Fresh is best, but the more greens the better. Our carb intake will be from vegetables only.

- The value of *adding lemon or lime and herbs and spices to your meal* should not be underestimated, for both taste and variety. Also, by alternating your seasonings, you can *avoid taste fatigue* – basically when your taste buds grow tired of a certain food because you've eaten it too often. It can also help you *avoid food intolerances.* If you've ingested a certain food too regularly, the body can also build up a resistance to it causing symptoms such as bloating after meals, cramping or feeling nauseous.

- Try to *avoid gluten* (see above).

- Avoid cereal, bread, rice, pasta, cookies etc.

- *Starchy foods* aren't forbidden provided they are gluten-free (such as sweet potato, rice and pasta), however, for the purpose of transforming the body, we mainly stick to fibrous carbohydrates. This includes all your plant-based vegies. This keeps insulin and therefore fat production low.

- Try and *keep dairy products to a minimum* as they can place an extra load on the digestive system. Unless you can get hold of unpasteurised, unhomogenised milk, I would use products from goats or try rice or almond milk.

- *Water intake* is essential, preferably filtered and drunk out of an aluminium or BPA-free plastic drink bottle. Try and drink at least 3–4 litres (100–135 fluid ounces) a day.

- *Minimise alcohol* as much as possible to avoid slowing down fat loss (see above).

- Try and *eat no later than 7.30 pm*. This is important for digestion and helps to wind the body down, ensuring good hormonal health.

- Try and include one *load meal or refuel day* a week (see above).

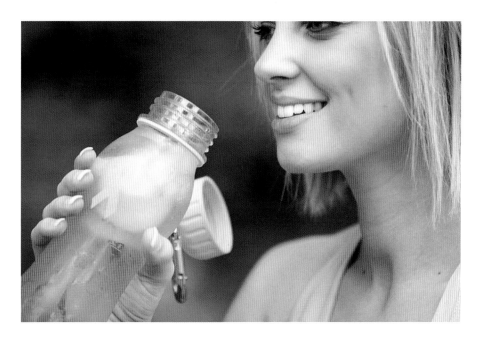

Water intake is essential, preferably filtered and drunk out of an aluminium or BPA-free plastic drink bottle. Try and drink at least 3–4 litres (100–135 fluid ounces) a day.

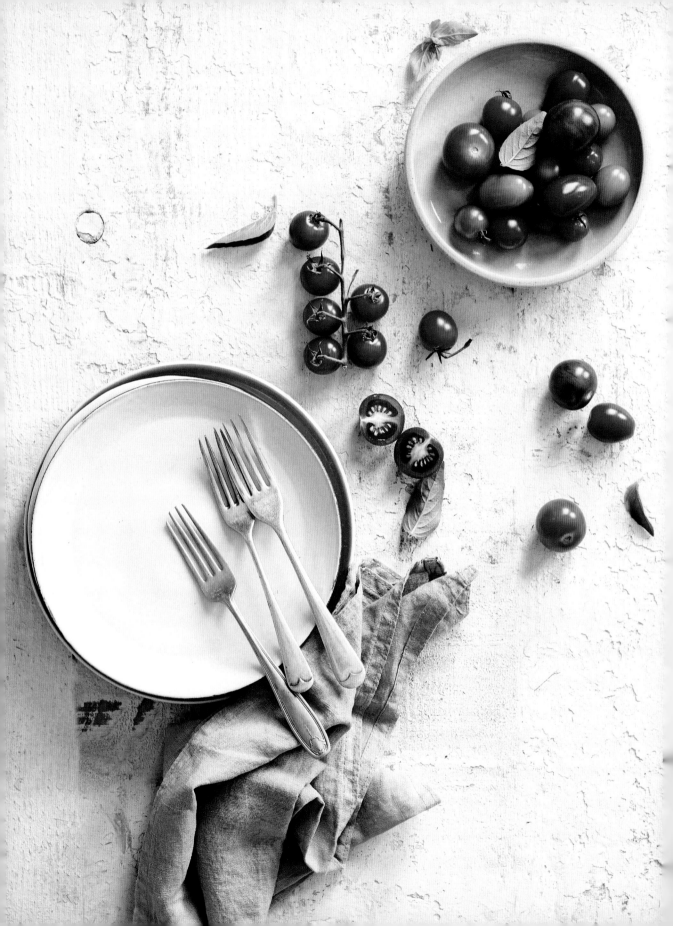

recipes
for a
healthy
lifestyle

The battle is won - and lost - at the dinner table.
Keep it clean and simple, shredders!

Turkey cups

Preparation: 10 mins

Cooking time: 10 mins

Serves: 2

Tip Grab yourself a silicon muffin tray for ease of removal.

Ingredients

8 eggs

handful of parsley, finely chopped

6 cherry tomatoes

6 slices of turkey

Method

Preheat oven to 200ºC (390ºF). Grease or line a muffin tray.

Crack eggs into a mixing bowl and whisk until fluffy.

Finely chop parsley and cut cherry tomatoes in half.

Add the parsley to the eggs. Whisk briskly (the more you whisk, the lighter and fluffier they will be).

Line six muffin holes with a slice of turkey and pour in the egg mix. Fill the cup to the top and place two cherry tomato halves on top of each turkey cup.

Place in a preheated oven for 10–12 minutes or until golden.

Serve immediately.

MACRONUTRIENTS
per serve

Protein 31.7g (1.1oz)

Fats   22.7g (0.8oz)

Carbs   3.2g   (0.1oz)

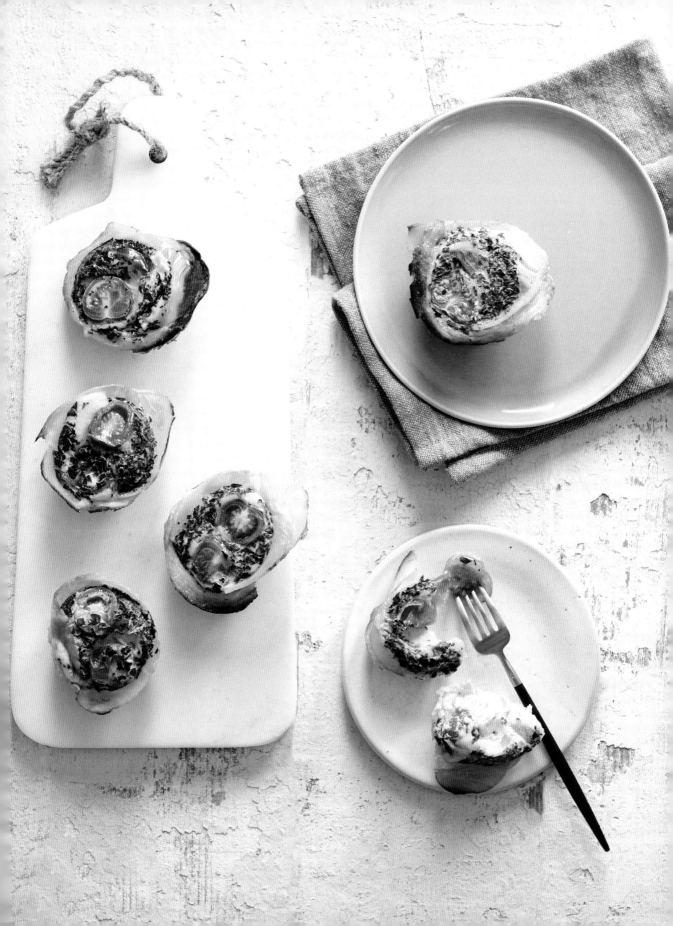

Brekky frittata

Preparation: 10 mins

Cooking time: 10 mins

Serves: 2

Ingredients

grapeseed oil

4 mushrooms, sliced thinly

½ onion, finely chopped

3 kale leaves, sliced thinly

5 eggs

freshly cracked pepper

handful of parsley, finely chopped

3 slices of ham, finely chopped

Method

Preheat oven to 180ºC (350ºF). Grease an oven-proof fry pan.

Drizzle some grapeseed oil into a pan and fry mushrooms and onion until soft. Add kale and toss for 30 seconds, then remove from heat and place in a bowl.

Crack the eggs into separate bowl and mix well. Season with pepper and add parsley and ham. Combine.

Return mixture to the pan and cook until the eggs start to set. Then place directly in the oven for approximately 8 minutes or until the egg has risen slightly and is cooked through.

Slice and serve.

MACRONUTRIENTS
per serve

Protein 25.2g (0.9oz)

Fats   19.5g (0.7oz)

Carbs   4.0g (0.1oz)

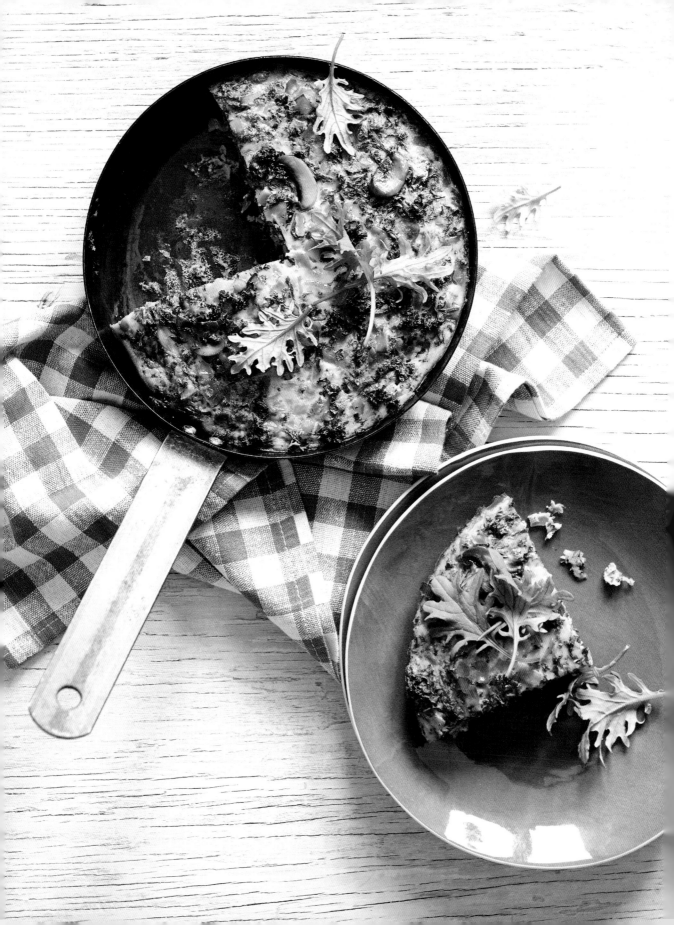

Healthy hash

Preparation: 10 mins

Cooking time: 20 mins

Serves: 4

Ingredients

2 tsp grapeseed oil

2 cloves of garlic, finely chopped

1 brown onion, finely chopped

500g (1.1lb) lean beef mince

60g (2oz) or small handful of pine nuts

50g (1.75oz) or large handful of baby spinach, finely chopped

½ bunch parsley, finely chopped

salt (iodised or Himalayan) and freshly cracked pepper

4 eggs

> ### MACRONUTRIENTS
> per serve
>
> Protein 37.0g (1.3oz)
> Fats   34.8g (1.2oz)
> Carbs   15.8g (0.6oz)

Method

Fill a medium size saucepan with water and bring to the boil, ready to soft poach the eggs.

Drizzle some grapeseed oil into a pan and caramelise garlic and onion. Add the beef mince and cook until brown, occasionally breaking it up with a wooden spoon.

Remove the cooked mince from the pan and place in a large mixing bowl. Add pine nuts, baby spinach and parsley. Season with salt and pepper and mix through.

Poach eggs by cracking over a skimmer (poaching tool) to drain off the outer egg white. Carefully place the remainder of the egg into the water. Repeat with the other eggs and leave to poach for 2 minutes or until the white is set.

Divide the meat into four bowls and place a poached egg on top of each one. Season to taste.

To eat, break the cooked egg and mix the yolk through the hash.

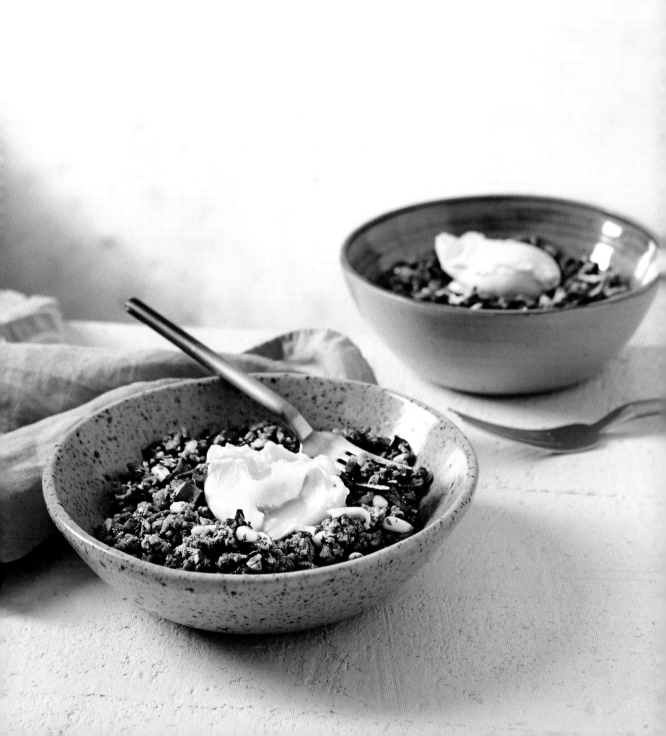

Mediterranean-style omelette

Preparation: 5 mins

Cooking time: 10 mins

Serves: 2

Ingredients

4 eggs

small bunch of chives, finely chopped

1 tsp grapeseed oil, plus extra for drizzling

3 slices of smoked chicken breast, roughly chopped

50g (1.75oz) feta, crumbled

8 semi-sundried tomatoes, roughly chopped

a handful kalamata olives, pitted and halved

150g (5.5oz) baby spinach

freshly squeezed lemon juice, to taste

freshly cracked pepper

Method

Crack eggs into a bowl and whisk until fluffy. Stir through chives.

Heat the oil in a non-stick frying pan, add the eggs and cook, swirling with a fork as they set. While the eggs are still slightly runny, add the chicken, feta, sundried tomatoes and olives evenly over the top. Fold the omelette in half and cook for one more minute or until cooked through.

Slide onto a plate and serve with baby spinach drizzled with lemon juice, a drizzle of grapeseed oil and freshly cracked black pepper

MACRONUTRIENTS
per serve

Protein 42.0g (1.5oz)

Fats   36.2g (1.3oz)

Carbs   18.0g (0.6oz)

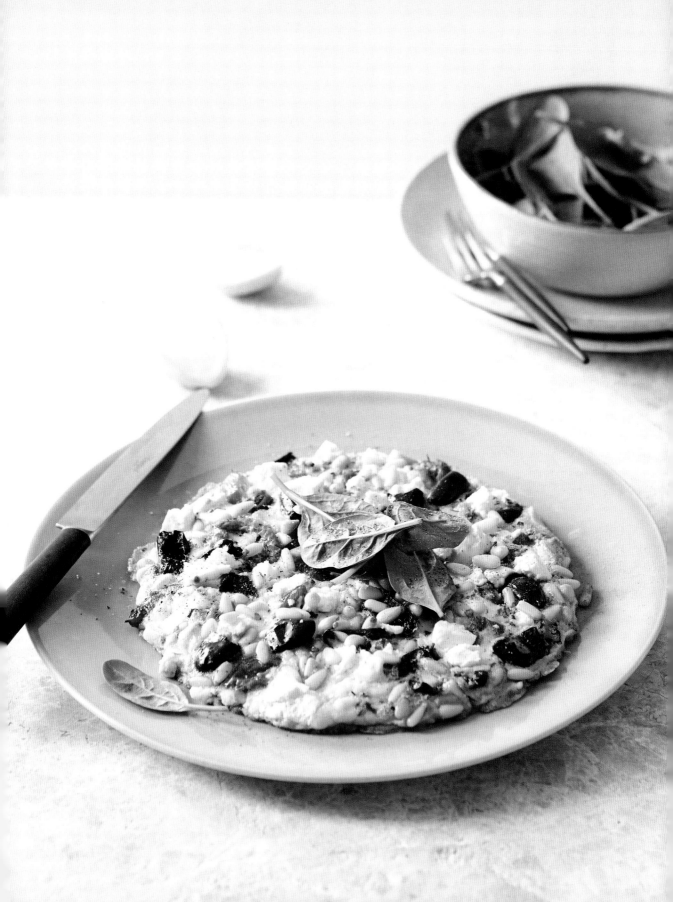

Classic scrambled eggs with salmon and dill

Preparation: 5 mins

Cooking time: 5 mins

Serves: 2

Ingredients

4 eggs plus 1 egg white

1 tsp olive oil

sprinkling of paprika

200g (7oz) smoked salmon, roughly chopped

small bunch dill, finely chopped

½ lemon, cut into quarters

Method

Crack the eggs into a bowl and whisk until fluffy.

Heat the olive oil in a non-stick frying pan over a medium heat and add the eggs. Stir continuously with a wooden spoon, removing from the heat while they are still slightly runny (they will continue to cook off the heat).

Divide the eggs between two plates, sprinkle with paprika, top with salmon and dill, and serve with a lemon wedge.

MACRONUTRIENTS
per serve

Protein 39.0g (1.4oz)

Fats   34.6g (1.2oz)

Carbs   12.2g (0.4oz)

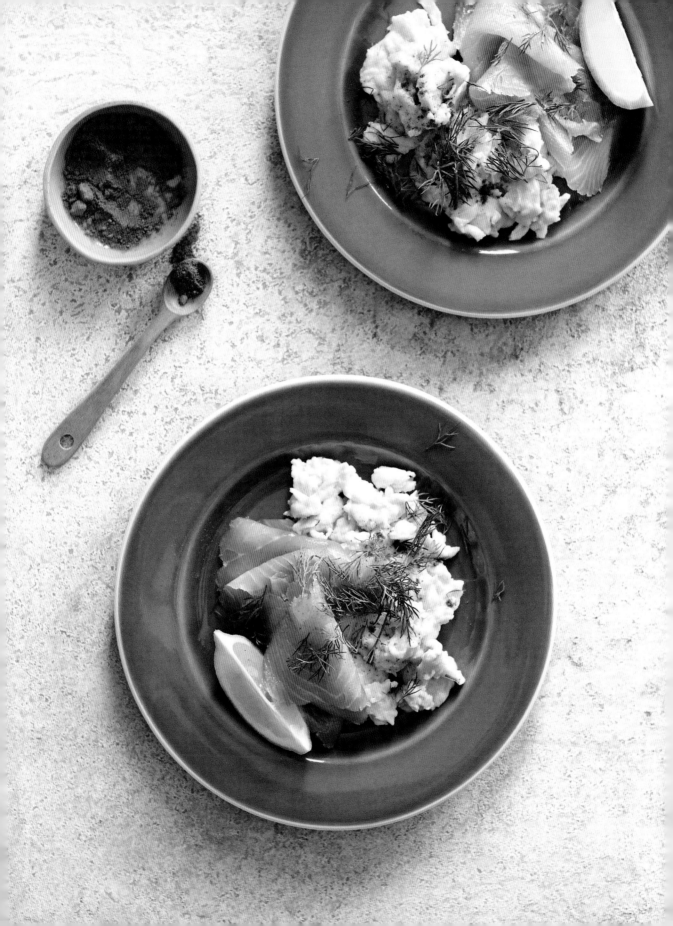

Savoury super-food bowl with poached egg

Preparation: 5 mins
(plus time to cook quinoa)

Cooking time: 20 mins

Serves: 2

Tip Also makes a great brunch dish.

Ingredients

½ bunch asparagus, ends snapped off

1 garlic clove, crushed

2 eggs

100g (3.5oz) haloumi, sliced into 1 cm pieces

150g (5.25oz) quinoa, cooked as per instructions on packet

handful of rocket

olive oil, to drizzle

salt (iodised or Himalayan) and freshly cracked pepper

sprinkle of paprika or cayenne

MACRONUTRIENTS
per serve

Protein 19.8g (0.7oz)

Fats   10.2g (0.4oz)

Carbs   18.2g (0.6oz)

Method

In a saucepan, bring enough water to a simmer to submerge the asparagus. Add the asparagus and garlic and cook for 2 minutes or until asparagus is bright green but still retains some crunch. Remove from the pan with tongs and cool under cold water to stop the cooking process. Set aside.

To soft poach eggs, fill a medium size saucepan with water and bring to the boil. Crack the eggs over a skimmer (poaching tool) to drain off the outer egg white. Carefully place the remainder of the egg into the water. Repeat with the other egg. Poach for 2 minutes or until the white is set.

Fry off haloumi in a non-stick frying pan over a medium heat until browned on both sides.

Fluff quinoa with a fork and divide between two bowls. Top with rocket, haloumi, asparagus and a poached egg. Drizzle with a little olive oil and sprinkle with salt, freshly cracked black pepper and paprika (or cayenne) to taste.

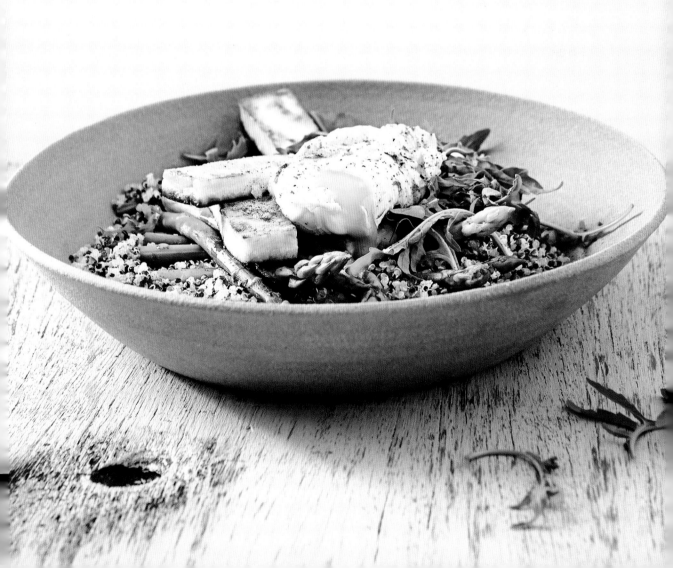

Turkey wraps with hummus spread

Preparation: 5 mins

Cooking time: nil

Serves: 1

Ingredients

100g (3.5oz) or 2 large turkey slices

1 tbsp hummus

1 carrot, diced

1 celery stick, diced

½ cucumber, diced

Method

Spread hummus over turkey slices. Place diced vegies over the hummus. Wrap the turkey into a roll. Enjoy.

MACRONUTRIENTS
per serve

Protein   22.1g (0.8oz)

Fats   4.6g (0.2oz)

Carbs   17.7g (0.6oz)

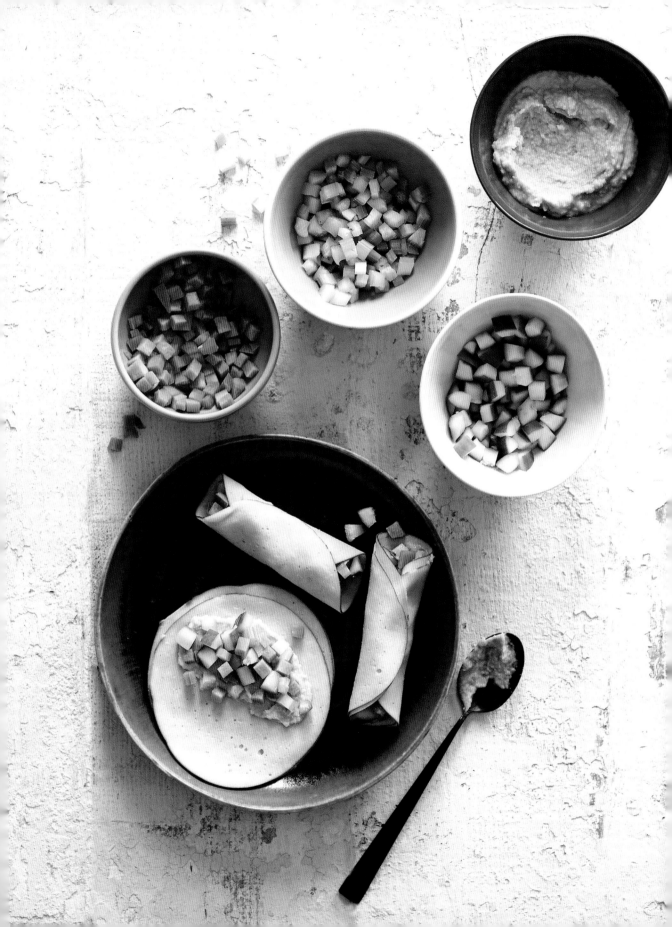

Egg boats

Preparation: 5 mins

Cooking time: 10 mins

Serves: 1

Ingredients

6 eggs

½ red onion, finely chopped

2 celery sticks, diced

juice of ½ a lemon

2 tsp of Dijon mustard

½ tsp of paprika

salt (iodised or Himalayan) and freshly cracked pepper

1 lebanese cucumber, sliced in ½ lengthways, seeds removed, to make a boat

2 tsp chives, finely chopped

Method

Place eggs in a medium size saucepan of water. Bring to the boil and simmer for 8 minutes.

Mix lemon juice, mustard, paprika, salt and pepper in a bowl. Add the onion and celery.

Run eggs under cold water and remove shells. Dice two whole eggs and two of the whites only (discard the yolks). Add to the bowl and mix together.

Spoon eggs into cucumber boats and sprinkle with chives.

MACRONUTRIENTS
per serve

Protein 30.3g   (1.1oz)

Fats   17.2g (0.6oz)

Carbs   8.8g (0.3oz)

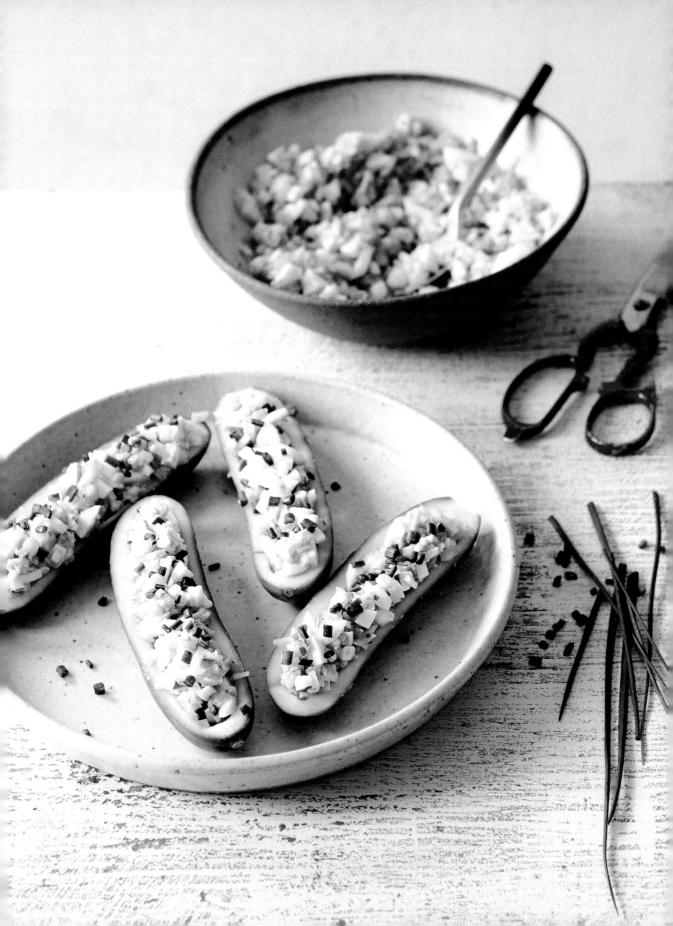

Capsicum egg cups

Preparation: 5 mins

Cooking time: 10 mins

Serves: 1

Ingredients

1 red capsicum

1 boiled egg

freshly cracked pepper

Method

Slice capsicum into four cheeks. Cut boiled egg into quarters and place one inside each capsicum cheek. Season with pepper.

MACRONUTRIENTS
per serve

Protein   6.5g (0.2oz)

Fats   4.3g (0.2oz)

Carbs   2.7g   (0.1oz)

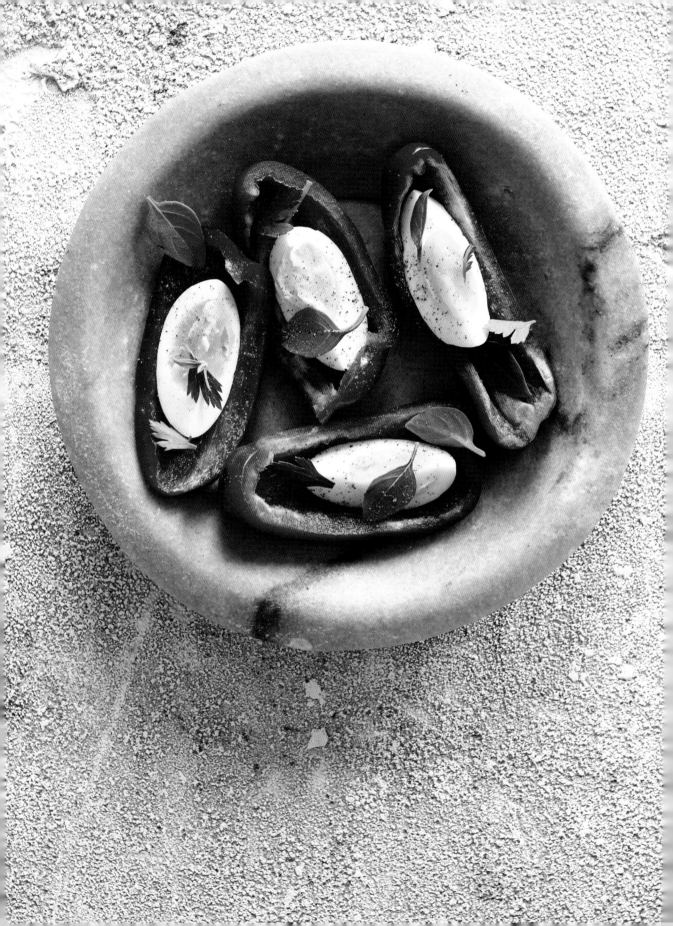

Prosciutto-wrapped asparagus

Preparation: 10 mins

Cooking time: 5 mins

Serves: 1

Tip Containing essential amino acids, asparagus is an important detoxifier but can also act as a diuretic, making your waistline smaller. If you have an event coming up, add it to a meal a day for seven days and notice your waistline diminish.

Ingredients

½ bunch of asparagus, ends snapped off

2-3 slices of prosciutto

grapeseed oil

Method

Bring a medium-sized frying pan of water to the boil. Place asparagus in boiling water and cook for 2 minutes or until bright green. Remove from the pan with tongs and cool under cold water to stop the cooking process.

Wrap the prosciutto around the asparagus sticks.

Empty water from the frying pan and dry. Drizzle a small amount of grapeseed oil into the pan and lightly fry the prosciutto-wrapped spears until golden.

Serve immediately.

MACRONUTRIENTS
per serve

Protein 14.7g (0.5oz)

Fats   6.1g   (0.2oz)

Carbs   1.4g (0.05oz)

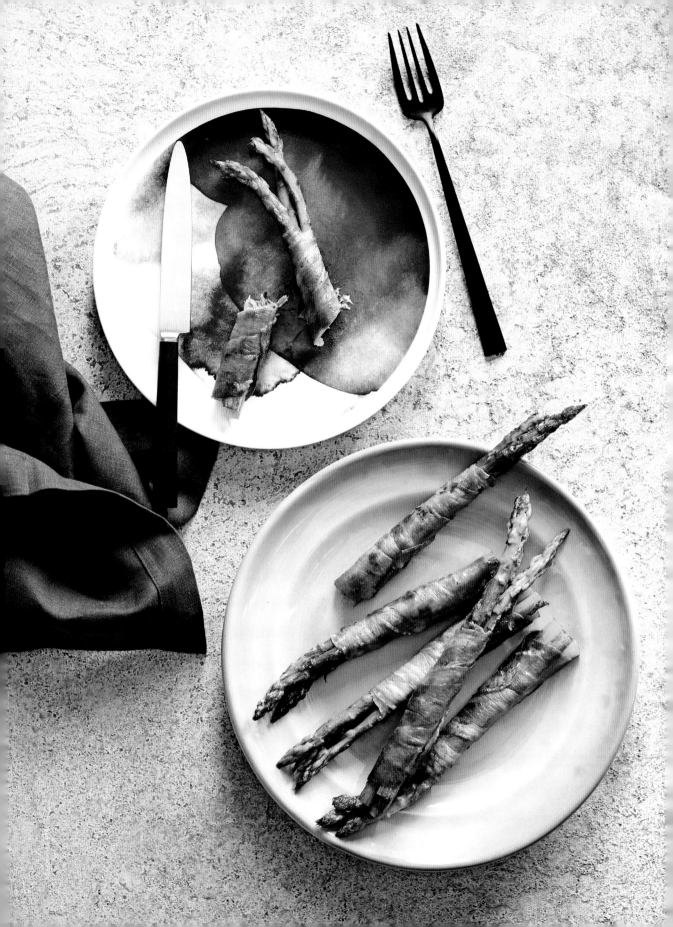

Spice-roasted mixed nuts

Preparation: 20 mins

Cooking time: 20 mins

Serves: 2

Ingredients

handful blanched almonds

handful cashews

½ tsp cayenne pepper

½ tsp cumin

½ tsp coriander (ground)

1 clove garlic, thinly sliced

zest of ½ lemon plus 1 tsp of lemon juice

iodised salt, to taste

Method

Preheat oven to 170ºC (340ºF).

Combine almonds, cashews, cayenne pepper, cumin, coriander, garlic, lemon zest and juice. Allow to stand for 15 minutes.

Transfer nuts onto a baking tray and sprinkle with a pinch of salt. Roast for around 20 minutes, stirring occasionally until nuts are dried out and golden.

Cool slightly and enjoy!

MACRONUTRIENTS
per serve

Protein 10.2g (0.4oz)

Fats   34.2g (1.2oz)

Carbs   3.6g   (0.1oz)

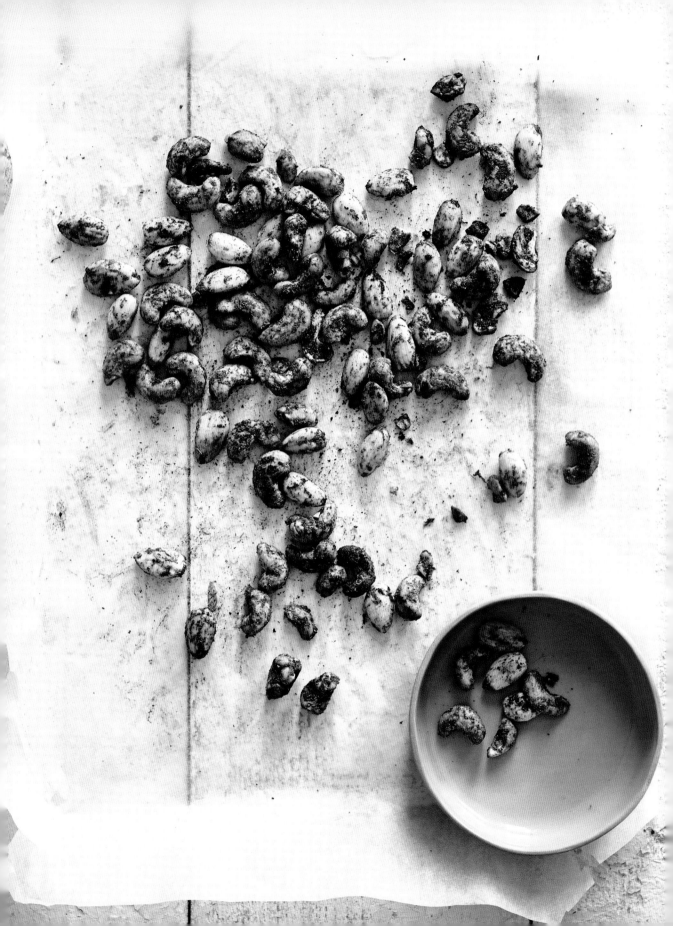

Avocado with marinated feta and crunchy sunflower seeds

Preparation: 5 mins

Cooking time: 5 mins

Serves: 2

Ingredients

50g (1.75oz) feta, crumbled

small bunch parsley, finely chopped

1 sprig rosemary, finely chopped

2 sprigs thyme, finely chopped

1 tsp good quality olive oil

freshly cracked pepper

1 avocado, halved

1 tsp balsamic vinegar

20g (0.75oz) sunflower seeds, toasted

Method

Combine feta with herbs and a drizzle of olive oil. Season with pepper and leave to marinate for a few minutes.

Drizzle avocado with a little balsamic vinegar, top with marinated feta and crunchy sunflower seeds. Enjoy!

MACRONUTRIENTS
per serve

Protein   9.8g (0.3oz)

Fats   28.0g (1.0oz)

Carbs   6.2g (0.2oz)

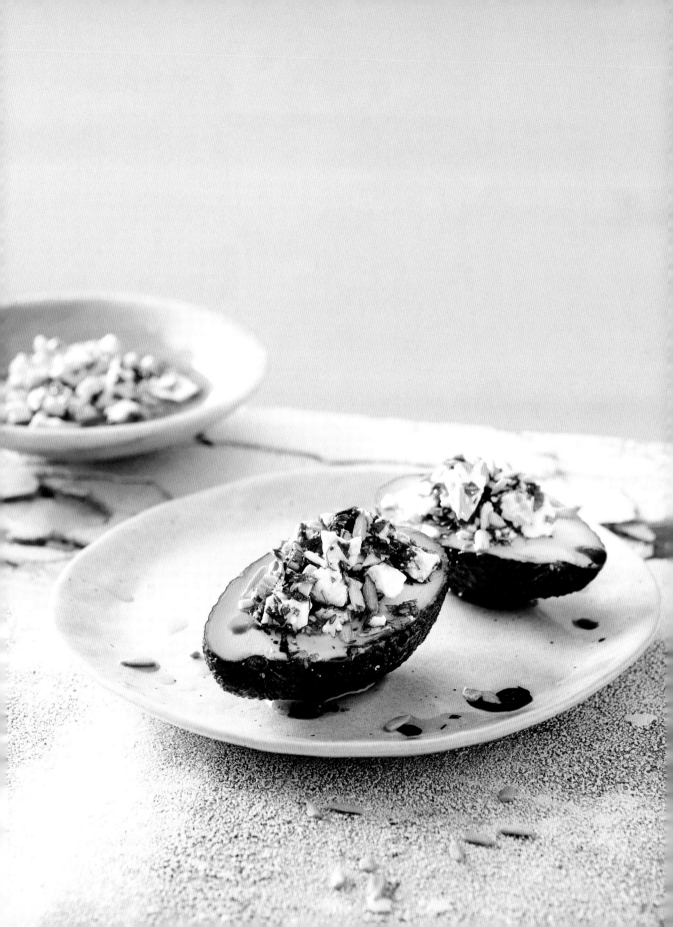

Poached chicken salad

Preparation: 10 mins

Cooking time: 25 mins

Serves: 4

Ingredients

600g (1.3lb) chicken breast

1 bunch of kale, stalks removed, finely sliced

2 medium radishes, finely sliced

100g (3.5oz) snow peas

60g (2oz) or small handful of almond flakes

50g (1.75oz) or large handful of parsley, finely chopped

Dressing

1 clove of garlic, crushed

juice of 1 lemon

½ cup of tahini (unhulled)

½ cup of water

salt (iodised or Himalayan) and freshly cracked pepper

Method

Bring a large pot of water to the boil. To poach the chicken, place in water and return to the boil. Lower the temperature and simmer for 20 minutes or until cooked through. Remove from the heat and let stand for 5 minutes.

Place kale, radishes and snow peas into a large salad bowl. Add almonds and parsley. Slice the chicken thinly and add to the salad. Toss.

Combine the dressing ingredients together in a small bowl and mix well. Drizzle over salad and serve.

MACRONUTRIENTS
per serve

Protein 48.7g (1.7oz)

Fats 19.6g (0.7oz)

Carbs 11.5g (0.4oz)

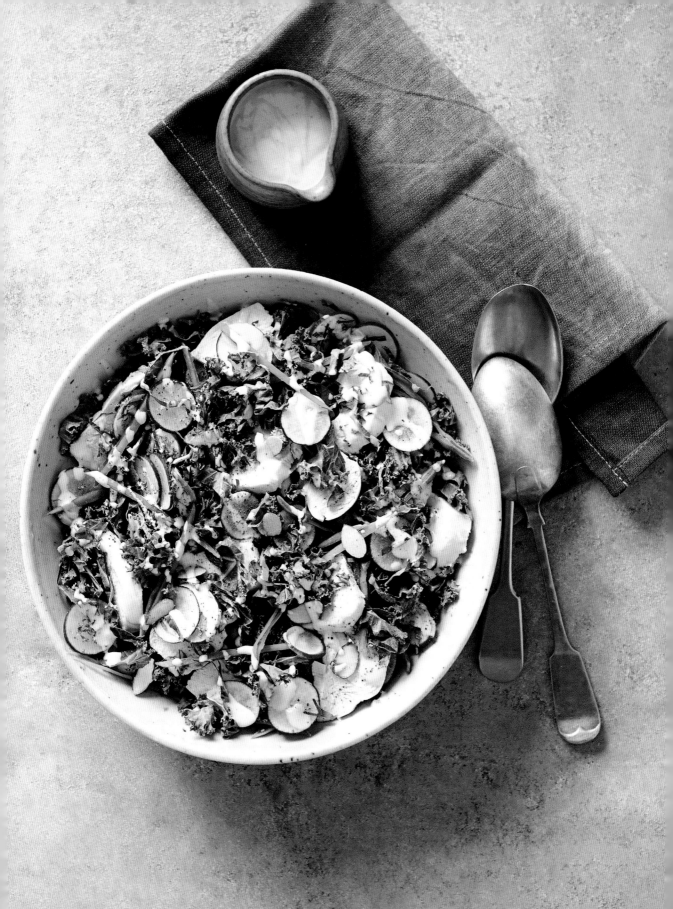

Chilli coriander squid

Preparation: 10 mins

Cooking time: 15 mins

Serves: 4

Tip Where possible, go organic. If this isn't possible, always rinse your vegies thoroughly with water. This will lessen the toxicity from pesticides and the impact it has on your body and its ability to burn fat.

Ingredients

2 red onions, peeled, halved and cut into wedges

4 tsp flaxseed oil, plus extra

1 tsp balsamic vinegar

2 chillies, finely chopped

1 bunch of coriander, finely chopped

600g (1.3lb) pre-cut squid rings or approximately 4 baby squid, scored and thinly sliced

1 punnet cherry tomatoes, halved

handful of kalamata olives

100g (3.5oz) rocket

50g (1.75oz) or large handful of parsley, roughly chopped

juice of ½ a lemon

Method

Preheat oven to 180ºC (350ºF). Line a baking tray with baking paper.

Place onion on a baking tray. Drizzle with half the flaxseed oil and balsamic vinegar and bake for 15 minutes. Set aside to cool.

Place chilli and coriander in a bowl with the squid. Toss together.

In a separate bowl, place cherry tomatoes, olives, rocket, parsley and onion.

Heat oil in pan and quickly toss squid for 2 minutes or until tender. Add to bowl with salad and toss. Drizzle with remaining flaxseed oil and lemon juice to serve.

MACRONUTRIENTS
per serve

Protein 28.7g (1.0oz)

Fats   8.3g (0.3oz)

Carbs   9.4g (0.3oz)

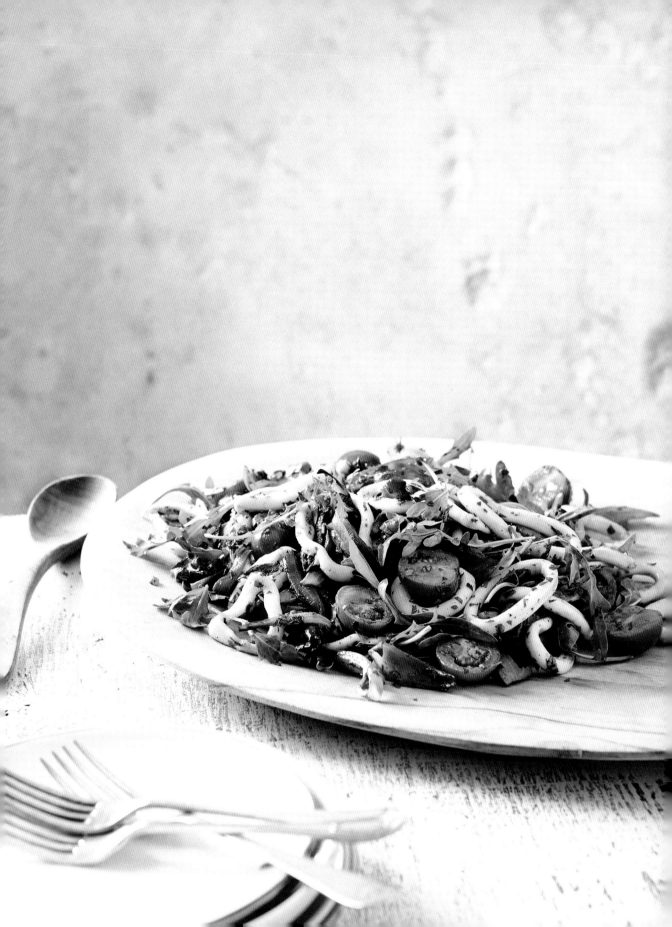

San choy bow

Preparation: 10 mins

Cooking time: 10 mins

Serves: 4

Ingredients

1 stick lemongrass, roughly chopped

2 large, red chillies, roughly chopped

3 large garlic cloves, roughly chopped

1 large knob of fresh ginger, roughly chopped

2 tbsp coconut oil, plus extra for frying

500g (1.1lb) lean pork mince

1 red capsicum, finely chopped

½ small bunch of mint, finely chopped

½ small bunch of coriander, finely chopped

4 kaffir limes leaves, thinly sliced

4 spring onions, thinly sliced

1 tbsp oyster sauce (gluten-free)

1 tsp fish sauce

juice of 2 limes

2 baby cos lettuce, ends removed and divided into cups

Method

Place lemongrass, chilli, garlic and ginger in a blender or food processor. Process until finely diced.

Heat oil in a pan and add the chilli mix. Stir for about 2 minutes or until fragrant.

Add pork mince and cook for about 5-6 minutes or until browned.

Add capsicum and stir through, cooking for a further 2 minutes.

Take pan off the heat and add the mint, coriander, kaffir lime leaves and spring onion, mixing well. Stir through the oyster sauce, fish sauce and lime juice.

Divide lettuce leaves between four plates and fill with pork mince.

Enjoy.

MACRONUTRIENTS
per serve

Protein 33.3g (1.2oz)

Fats 14.1g (0.5oz)

Carbs 9.8g (0.3oz)

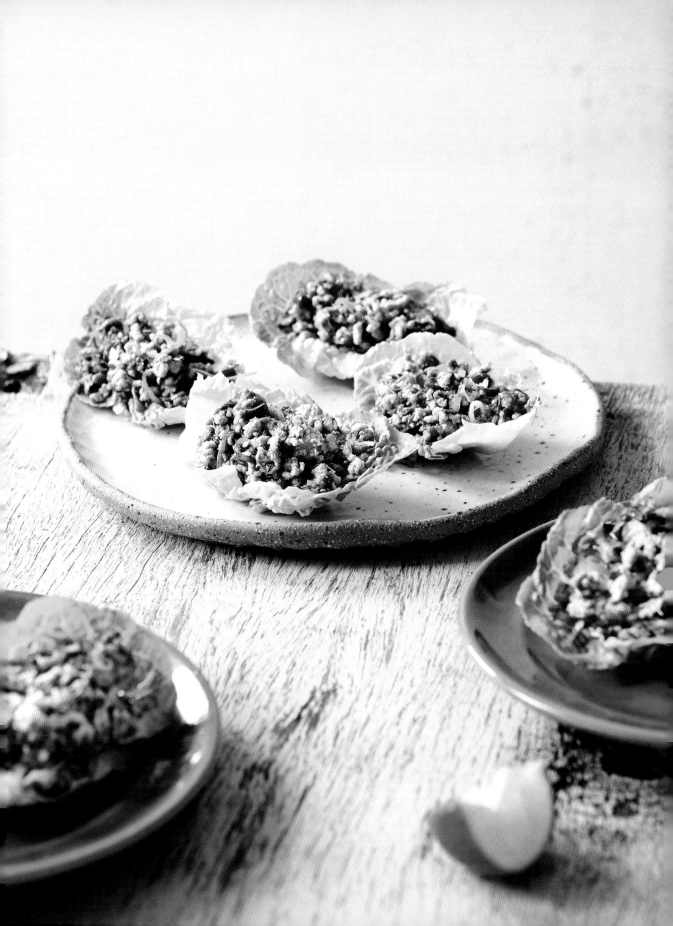

Turkey rissoles

Preparation: 10 mins

Cooking time: 15 mins

Serves: 4

Ingredients

2 tsp grapeseed oil

500g (1.1lb) turkey mince

1 brown onion, finely diced

2 garlic cloves, finely chopped

¼ bunch parsley, finely chopped

salt (iodised or Himalayan) and freshly cracked pepper

1 tsp ground fennel seeds

½ tsp ground coriander seeds

½ tsp smoked paprika

1 tsp flaxseed oil

2 tbsp of quinoa crumbs (gluten free)

1 egg yolk

Salsa

¼ cup pitted kalamata olives

1 cucumber, finely diced

1 tomato, finely diced

2 tsp flaxseed oil

juice of 1 large lemon

freshly cracked pepper

Method

Preheat oven to 180ºC (350ºF).

Grease an oven-proof frying pan with grapeseed oil.

Place turkey, onion, garlic and parsley in a mixing bowl and season. Add ground fennel and coriander, paprika and quinoa crumbs. Mix together well.

Using hands, roll mixture into balls.

Place balls into frying pan, pressing down slightly to flatten and brown for 3 minutes on each side. Then place in oven for 10 minutes to cook through.

Combine ingredients for salsa. Toss with flaxseed oil, lemon juice and pepper.

When cooked, place turkey rissoles on a plate and pour salsa over the top.

MACRONUTRIENTS
per serve

Protein 28.6g (1.0oz)

Fat   10.2g (0.4oz)

Carbs   8.2g (0.3oz)

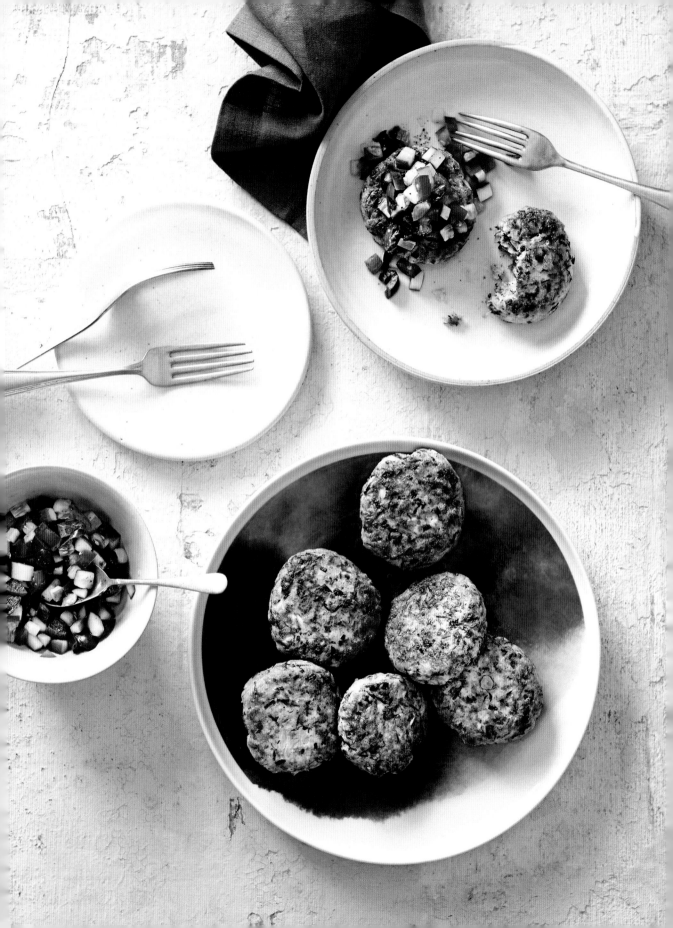

Shaved cucumber salad with raw kale pesto and mini pepper meatballs

Preparation: 15 mins

Cooking time: 20 mins

Serves: 2

Ingredients

250g (9oz) lean beef mince

1 egg, lightly whisked

1 brown onion, finely chopped

1 clove garlic, crushed, plus 1 clove extra, roughly chopped

½ green chilli, finely chopped

1 tsp freshly cracked pepper, plus extra

salt (iodised or Himalayan)

handful of kale

30g (1oz) pine nuts, toasted

2 tsp pumpkin seed oil

½ lemon, zested and juiced

2 cucumbers, shaved with a vegetable peeler, sprinkled with salt and placed in sieve over sink to remove excess water

200g (7oz) cherry tomatoes, halved

2 spring onions, finely chopped

MACRONUTRIENTS
per serve

Protein 31.8g   (1.1oz)

Fats   12.4g (0.4oz)

Carbs   10.2g (0.4oz)

Method

Preheat oven to 220°C (430°F). Line a small baking tray with baking paper.

For the meatballs, combine beef, egg, onion, garlic, chilli and 1 teaspoon pepper in a large bowl. Season with salt to taste.

Shape into 12 mini meatballs and arrange on baking tray. Place on the middle rack of the oven and cook for approximately 15-20 minutes, or until the meatballs are brown and cooked through.

Meanwhile, pulse kale, pine nuts, extra garlic, pumpkin seed oil, lemon juice and zest in a food processor until smooth. (If the mixture looks too dry, just add a little water.) Remove to a bowl, season with a little salt and pepper and set aside.

Remove meatballs from oven and allow to cool slightly.

Divide cucumber into serving bowls and top with dollops of pesto, meatballs, cherry tomatoes and spring onions.

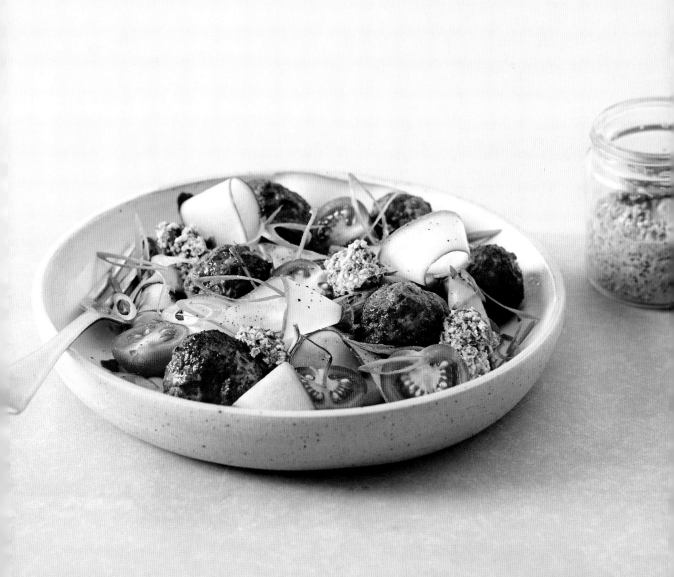

Quick and spicy turkey stir-fry

Preparation: 15 mins

Cooking time: 15 mins

Serves: 2

Ingredients

For the paste:

2 cloves of garlic, roughly chopped

½ red chilli, roughly chopped

5 cm piece of ginger, roughly chopped

½ lime, zested and juiced

1 lemongrass stalk, roughly chopped

1 brown onion, roughly chopped

1 tsp coconut oil

250g (9oz) turkey breast, diced

handful green beans, trimmed and halved

½ head broccoli, chopped into florets

1 red capsicum, cut into cubes

1 carrot, peeled and finely sliced

1 tbsp reduced fat coconut milk

small bunch coriander, roughly chopped

2 tsp cashew nuts, toasted and roughly chopped

Method

To make the paste, combine garlic, chilli, ginger, lime, lemongrass and onion in a food processor and pulse until smooth. (If the mixture looks too dry, just add a little water.)

Heat the oil in the wok. Add the turkey and brown on all sides. Set aside.

Add the paste to the pan and fry off until fragrant. Add the vegetables and stir-fry for approximately 5-8 minutes.

Add the browned turkey and coconut milk. Fry for another 3 minutes or until the turkey is cooked through but the vegies still have a bit of crunch to them.

Divide stir-fry between two plates and top with fresh coriander and cashews.

MACRONUTRIENTS
per serve

Protein 31.8g (1.1oz)

Fats   18.0g (0.6oz)

Carbs   14.6g (0.5oz)

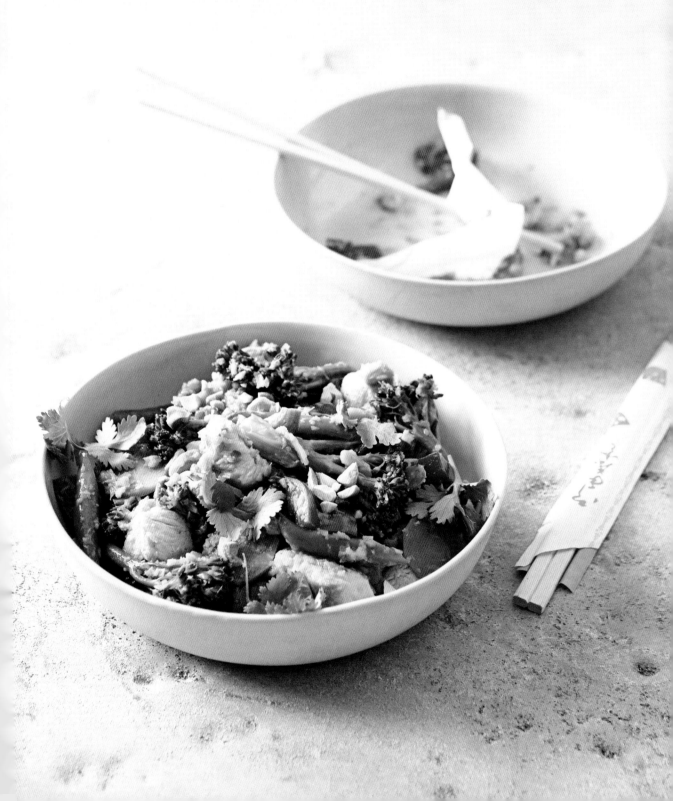

Lemon basil chicken in a bag

Preparation: 10 mins

Cooking time: 25 mins

Serves: 4

Ingredients

4 chicken breasts

grease-proof paper, 4 lengths x 70 cm

salt (iodised or Himalayan) and freshly cracked pepper

1 bunch asparagus, ends snapped off, each spear cut in half

1 bunch broccolini, trimmed and each floret cut in half

150g (5.5oz) sugar snap peas, destringed

4 sprigs basil

4 tsp flaxseed oil

2 lemons, 1 juiced and 1 thinly sliced

Method

Preheat oven to 200ºC (390ºF).

Place a chicken breast about halfway along each piece of baking paper and season.

Divide the greens evenly and lay over each piece of chicken. Top with basil leaves.

Drizzle a quarter of the flaxseed oil and the lemon juice onto each chicken breast. Top with sliced lemon.

Fold baking paper over the top of chicken and start pinching edges towards the chicken to create a bag.

Place on oven tray and cook for 25 minutes. Take extra care when unwrapping as steam will escape from the parcel. Serve immediately.

MACRONUTRIENTS
per serve

Protein 43.8g (1.5oz)

Fats   10.3g (0.4oz)

Carbs   8.6g (0.3oz)

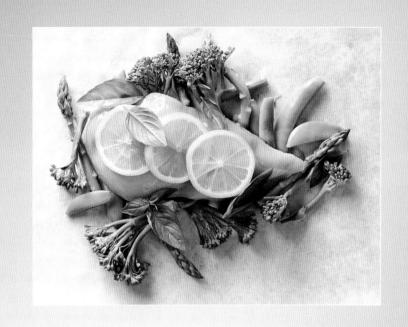

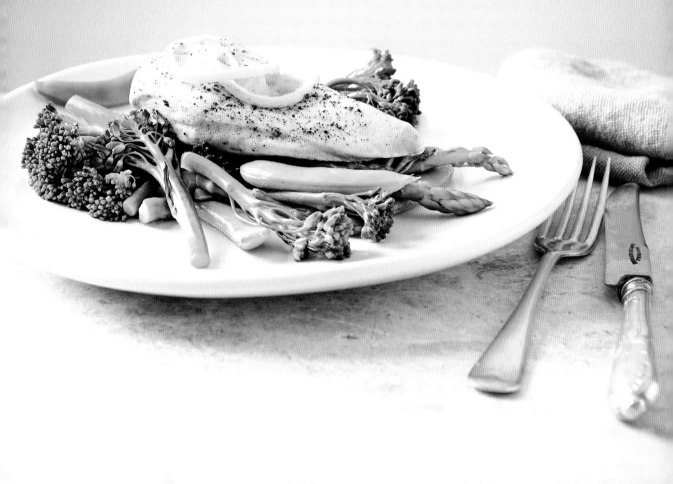

Clean spaghetti bolognese

Preparation: 15 mins

Cooking time: 15 mins

Serves: 4

Ingredients

1 tsp of extra virgin olive oil

1 brown onion, finely diced

2 celery sticks, finely diced

2 cloves of garlic, finely chopped

500g (1.1lb) beef mince

700g (1.5lb) bottle tomato passata

½ bunch broccolini, trimmed and each floret cut into 1 cm pieces

½ bunch asparagus, ends snapped off, each spear cut into 1 cm pieces

1 tbsp balsamic vinegar

salt (iodised or Himalayan) and freshly cracked pepper

2 zucchinis, made into spaghetti with a Betty Bossi (see below)

few sprigs of basil, leaves torn

Method

Place oil in a saucepan and add onion, celery and garlic. Cook until onion is golden. Add mince and stir until brown.

Stir in passata and simmer for 3 minutes, then add broccolini and asparagus.

Add vinegar and season. Leave to simmer on a low/medium heat for 15 minutes.

Just before you are ready to serve up, cook the zucchini spaghetti in the microwave for 30 seconds or until tender. Divide among four plates and top with bolognese sauce and some basil leaves.

Betty Bossi Vegetable Twister
The Betty Bossi is a fun and easy way of creating a spaghetti look and texture without the carbs and gluten. Great to make with kids.

MACRONUTRIENTS
per serve

Protein 35.3g (1.2oz)

Fats   14.8g (0.5oz)

Carbs   14.5g (0.5oz)

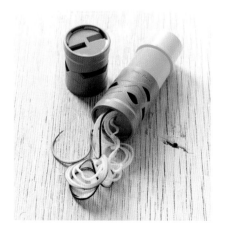

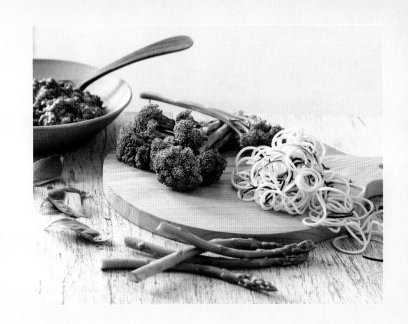

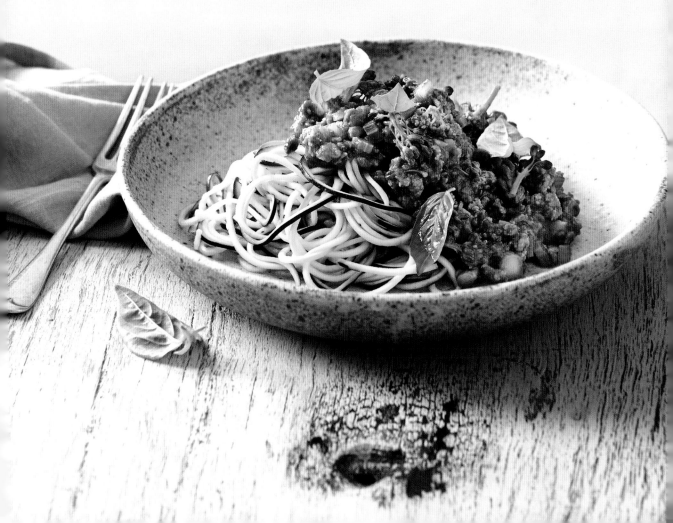

Prawn skewers

Preparation: 10 mins

Cooking time: 15 mins

Serves: 4

Ingredients

8 wooden skewers, soaked in water
for 45 minutes

2 tsp olive oil, plus extra

2 tsp ground cumin

500g (1.1lb) green prawns, peeled and
deveined

1 red capsicum, cut into 2 cm dice

1 green capsicum, cut into 2 cm dice

2 red onions, cut into 2 cm dice

2 zucchini, cut into 2 cm dice

200g (7oz) mushroom cups, halved

Method

Place the prawns in a bowl. Drizzle over
oil and sprinkle over cumin, mixing well
so that the prawns are covered well.

Thread the prawns and vegetables onto
the skewers.

Heat oil in large pan and place skewers
on to cook. Turn every so often until
vegetables are golden and prawns
are done.

MACRONUTRIENTS
per serve

Protein 31.8g   (1.1oz)

Fats   7.1g   (0.3oz)

Carbs   9.6g   (0.3oz)

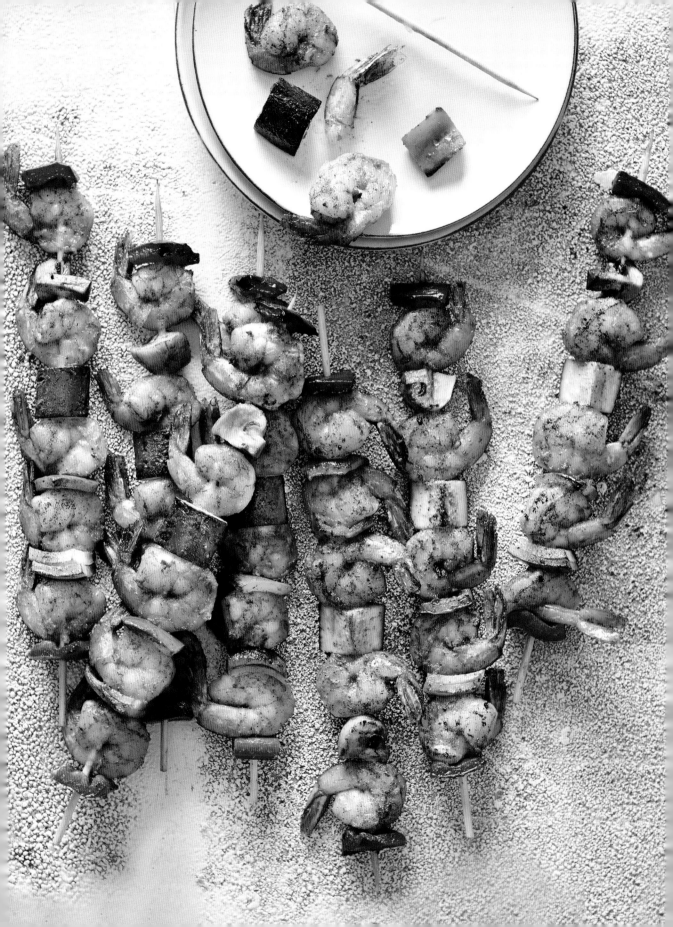

Red snapper and green beans with almonds

Preparation: 5 mins

Cooking time: 10 mins

Serves: 4

Ingredients

600g (1.3lb) red snapper steak, cut into 4 pieces of similar size

400g (14oz) green beans

1 tsp extra virgin olive oil, plus extra

1 lemon, sliced, to serve

salt (iodised or Himalayan) and freshly cracked pepper

60g (2oz) or small handful of almond flakes, optional

Method

Fill a medium saucepan that fits a bamboo steamer $\frac{1}{3}$ full with water and bring to the boil.

Meanwhile, line the steamer with baking paper. Place the green beans in the steamer and lay fish fillets over the top. Drizzle with olive oil and then lay lemon slices on top of fish. Season and put the lid on the steamer.

Place steamer over boiling water, making sure the steamer is not touching the boiling water.

Cook for 10-12 minutes depending on thickness of fish. Test by piercing fish with a sharp knife. It is done when the fish flakes and is opaque.

Carefully remove the steamer. Divide the fish, beans and lemon between four plates and sprinkle over the almonds, if using.

Serve.

MACRONUTRIENTS
per serve

Protein 41.3g (1.5oz)

Fats   15.2g (0.5oz)

Carbs   4.5g (0.2oz)

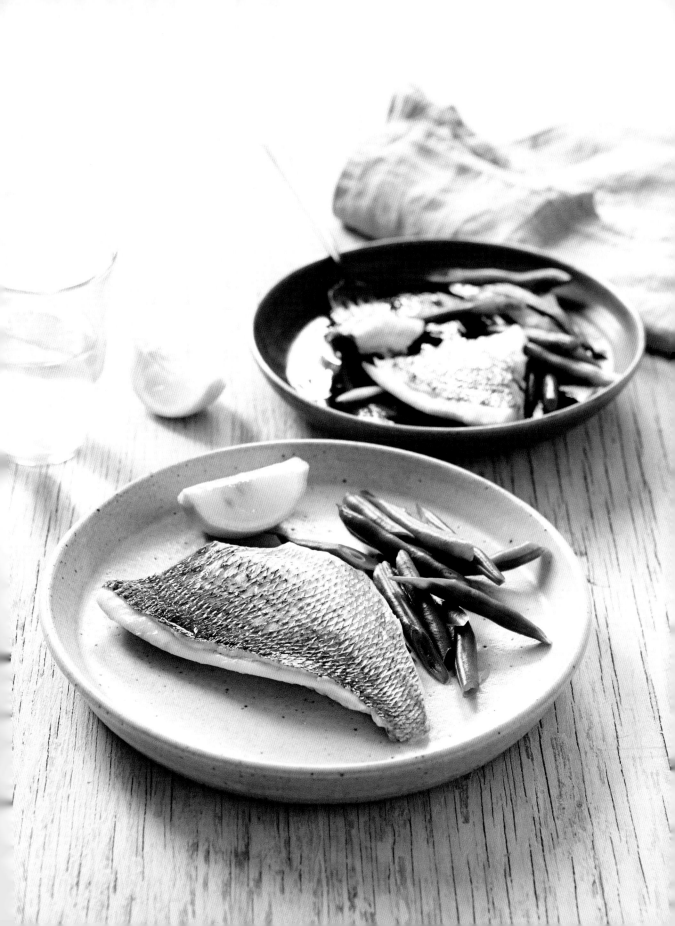

Whole seabass baked with citrus and swiss chard

Preparation: 10 mins

Cooking time: 40 mins

Serves: 2

Ingredients

2 small seabass, scaled and gutted (you can ask your fishmonger to do this)

small bunch parsley, finely chopped

2 cloves of garlic, crushed

1 fennel bulb, finely sliced

½ lemon, finely sliced

½ orange, finely sliced

handful kalamata olives, pitted and halved

1 tsp grapeseed oil, plus 1 tsp extra

salt (iodised or Himalayan) and freshly cracked pepper

250g (9oz) swiss chard, trimmed, white stems removed and cut into thin matchsticks, leaves roughly chopped

1 brown onion, finely sliced

> **MACRONUTRIENTS**
> per serve
>
> Protein 42.0g (1.5oz)
> Fats   8.6g (0.3oz)
> Carbs   18.0g (0.6oz)

Method

Preheat oven to 200°C (390°F). Rinse and dry the fish.

Mix the parsley, garlic, fennel, lemon and orange together. Use half of the mixture to stuff the cavity of the fish and place the remaining mixture with the olives on the bottom of a roasting tin.

Place the fish on top, drizzle with 1 teaspoon of grapeseed oil, season with some salt and pepper. Bake on the middle rack of the oven for about 30 minutes or until the fish is cooked through.

In the meantime, blanch the chard stems in boiling, salted water for 1-2 minutes, or until just soft. Remove from the pan with tongs and set aside. Blanch the green leaves in the boiling, salted water for 4-5 minutes, then drain well.

Heat the remaining teaspoon of grapeseed oil in a non-stick frying pan and fry off onion until soft. Add the swiss chard and fry for another 1-2 minutes or until heated through.

Divide the chard between two plates and top with fennel, olives and seabass.

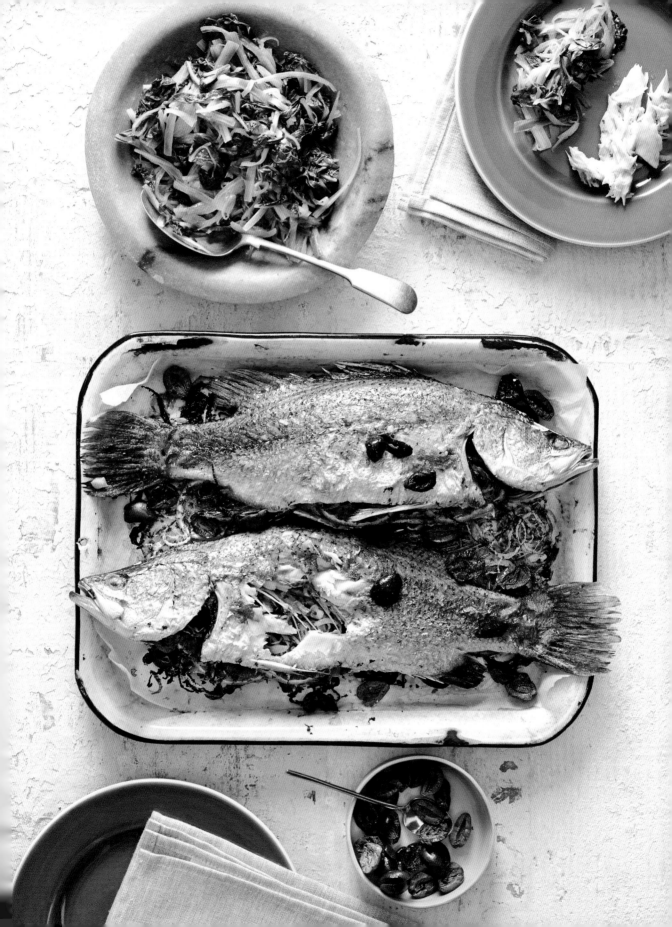

Moroccan steak salad

Preparation: 10 mins

Cooking time: 10 mins

Serves: 2

Ingredients

1 eggplant, diced

1 tsp olive oil, plus 1 tsp extra

1 tsp harissa

250g (9oz) cherry tomatoes, halved

200g (7oz) lean steaks

1 tsp cumin

1 tsp smoked paprika

½ lemon, juiced

100g (3.5oz) rocket

small bunch of mint, roughly chopped

small bunch of parsley, roughly chopped

handful baby spinach

1 pomegranate, halved and beaten gently over a large bowl with a wooden spoon to loosen the seeds.

Method

Mix eggplant with 1 tsp of olive oil and fry off in a non-stick pan until soft. Combine with harissa and tomatoes in a large bowl and set aside.

Fry steaks in a non-stick frying pan for around 3 minutes per side for medium-rare. Remove from the pan, cover with aluminum foil and leave to rest for a couple of minutes.

Combine the remaining olive oil with cumin, smoked paprika and lemon juice. Add to the eggplant with the rocket, mint, parsley and spinach and toss to combine.

Thinly slice the steaks and arrange on top of the salad, scatter with pomegranate seeds and enjoy!

MACRONUTRIENTS
per serve

Protein 33.2g (1.2oz)

Fats 14.2g (0.5oz)

Carbs 13.6g (0.5oz)

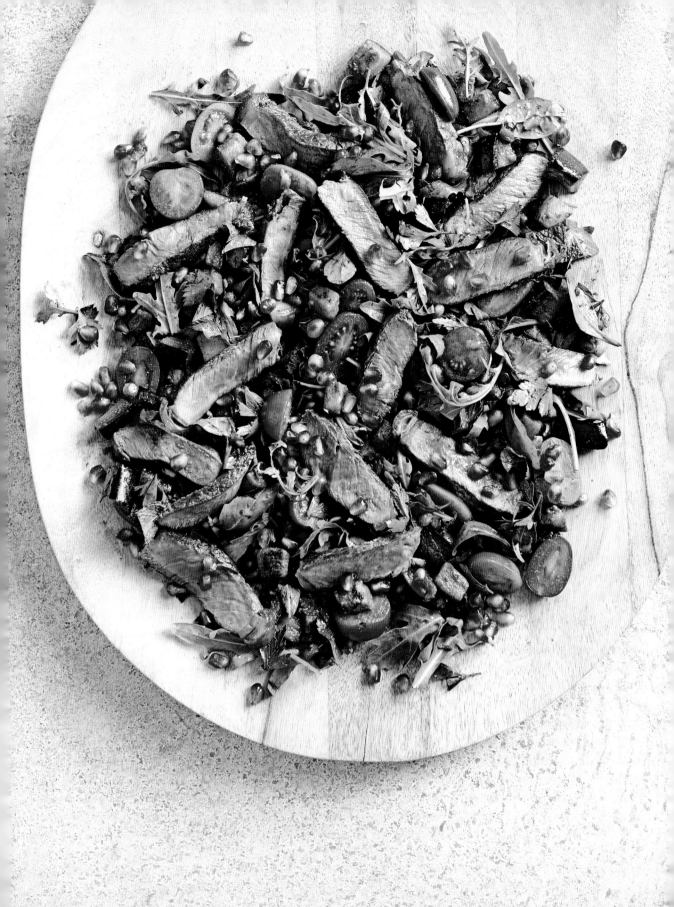

Cacao protein muffins

Preparation: 5 mins

Cooking time: 25 mins

Makes: 12 muffins (1 per serve)

> *Tip* Grab yourself a silicon muffin tray for ease of removal.

Method

1 cup quinoa flour

1 cup almond meal

½ cup cacao powder

1 tsp baking powder (gluten free)

1 scoop protein powder, preferably WPI (whey protein isolate)

½ cup coconut oil

⅔ cup almond milk

½ cup agave syrup

1 tsp vanilla extract

2 eggs

Almond icing

3 tbsp almond spread

1 tbsp cacao powder

⅛ teaspoon of stevia

3 tbsp hot water, more if needed

cacao nibs, if desired

Ingredients

Preheat oven to 180ºC (350ºF). Grease a muffin tray.

Sift quinoa flour, almond meal, cacao powder and baking powder into a bowl. Add protein powder, coconut oil, almond milk, agave and vanilla and mix well.

In a separate bowl, crack both eggs and whisk until combined. Add to the mixing bowl and combine all the ingredients until smooth.

Spoon mixture into a muffin tray and bake in the oven for 20 minutes. Remove and stand for 5 minutes, then remove from muffin tray. Cool.

Meanwhile, to make the almond icing, mix all the ingredients in a small bowl and stir until smooth. Spread over cool muffins.

> **MACRONUTRIENTS per muffin**
>
> Protein   11.4g (0.4oz)
>
> Fats   24.7g (0.9oz)
>
> Carbs   8.2g   (0.3oz)

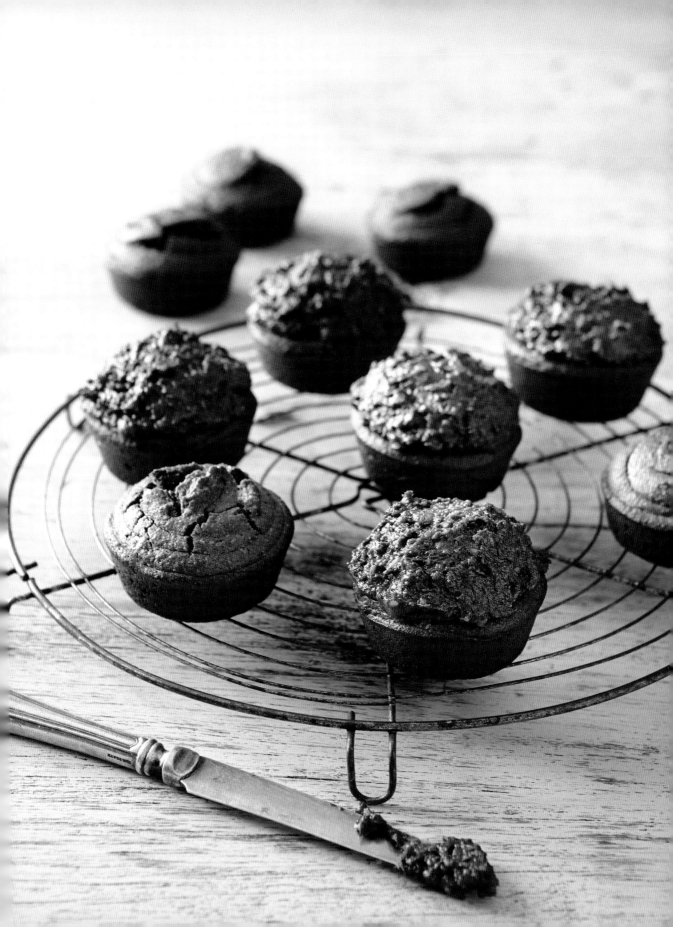

Protein pancakes

Preparation: 10 mins

Cooking time: 15 mins

Serves: 4 (2 pancakes per serve)

Tip Keep the already-made pancakes in a warm oven so they don't lose their heat while the others are being cooked.

Ingredients

2 eggs

1 scoop protein powder, preferably WPI (whey protein isolate)

½ cup gluten-free flour

¼ cup almond meal

½ tsp baking powder

2 tsp applesauce

½ cup almond milk

¼ cup coconut oil

2 tbsp chia seeds

1 cup of frozen blueberries

¾ cup Greek yoghurt to serve

Method

Crack eggs into the food processor and mix until light and fluffy. Add all the other ingredients except the chia seeds and mix until smooth. Gently fold the chia seeds through the mixture.

Heat a non-stick pan on a low/medium heat and add coconut oil.

Place a large spoonful of pancake mix into the pan and cook for approximately 2 minutes on each side or until golden brown. (Mixture should make 8 pancakes.)

Divide pancakes between four plates and serve with blueberries and Greek yoghurt.

MACRONUTRIENTS
per serve

Protein 22.8g (0.8oz)

Fats 30.8g (1.1oz)

Carbs 28.9g (1.0oz)

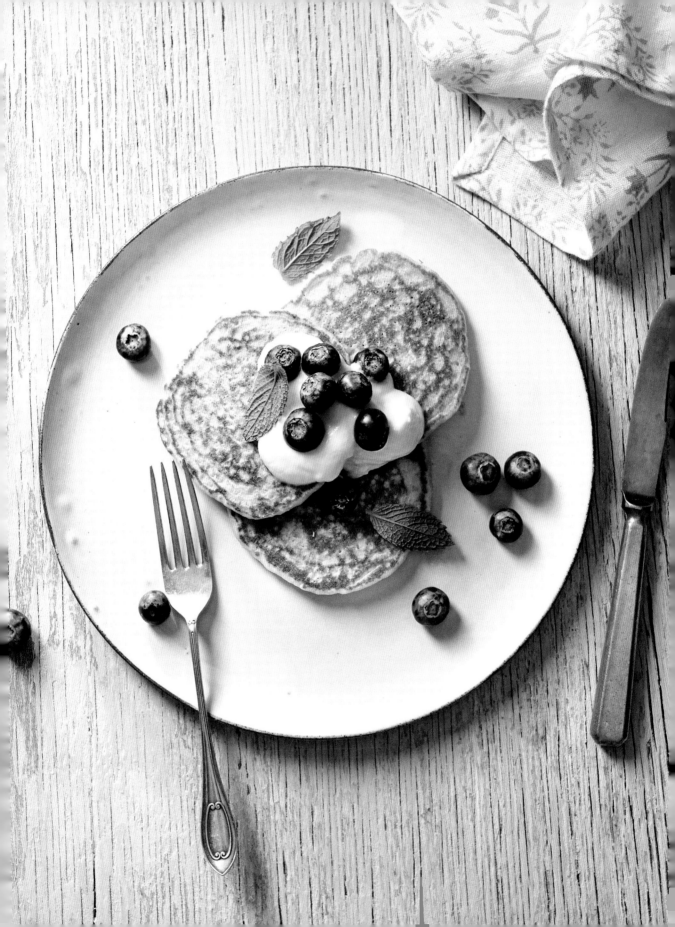

Protein balls

Preparation: 10 mins

Cooking time: nil

Makes: 12 balls

Serves: 4 (3 balls per serve)

Ingredients

1 cup dried apricots

$\frac{1}{2}$ cup dried craisins

$\frac{1}{2}$ cup goji berries

1 cup almonds

$\frac{1}{2}$ cup brazil nuts

$1\frac{1}{2}$ cup coconut flakes

$1\frac{1}{2}$ scoops vanilla protein powder,
preferably WPI (whey protein isolate)

$\frac{1}{4}$ cup agave syrup

$\frac{1}{2}$ cup desiccated coconut, for rolling

Method

Place apricots, craisins and goji berries into a food processor and mix on a high speed until it comes together in a ball.

Add the almonds, brazil nuts, coconut flakes, protein powder and agave syrup. Mix for approximately 2-3 minutes or until mixture comes together.

With lightly wet hands, roll into balls and coat with desiccated coconut.

Place in a container and refrigerate. Will keep for 3 days.

MACRONUTRIENTS
per serve (3 balls)

Protein   24.1g   (0.9oz)

Fats   56.6g   (2.0oz)

Carbs   65.0g   (2.3oz)

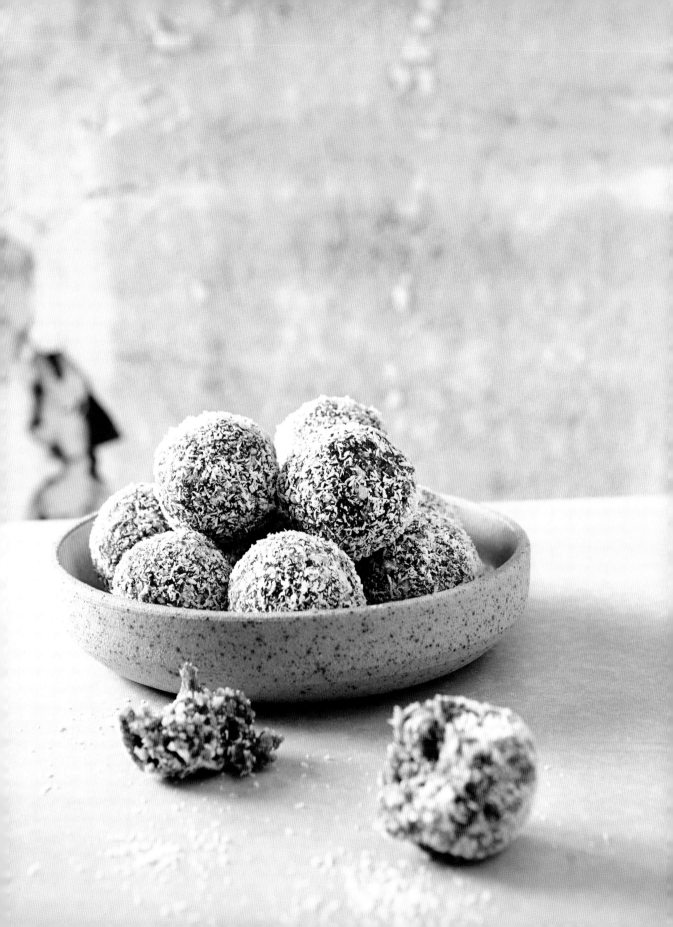

Chocolatey amaranth crumbles

Preparation: 5 mins

Cooking time: 10 mins (plus cooling time)

Makes: 12 puffs

Ingredients

200g (7oz) dark chocolate (at least 70% cocoa)

100g (3.5oz) roasted almonds (unsalted), roughly chopped

1½ tbsp coconut oil

125g (4.5oz) puffed amaranth

Method

Break chocolate into small pieces and place into a medium-sized pan on the lowest heat.

When the chocolate starts to melt, add the almonds and the coconut oil. Take the pan off the heat, add the amaranth and stir well until combined. Spoon into muffin cases (this can get a bit messy).

Place in fridge until set and store in an airtight container.

MACRONUTRIENTS
per serve

Protein 10.2g (0.4oz)

Fats   48.0g (1.7oz)

Carbs   62.8g (2.2oz)

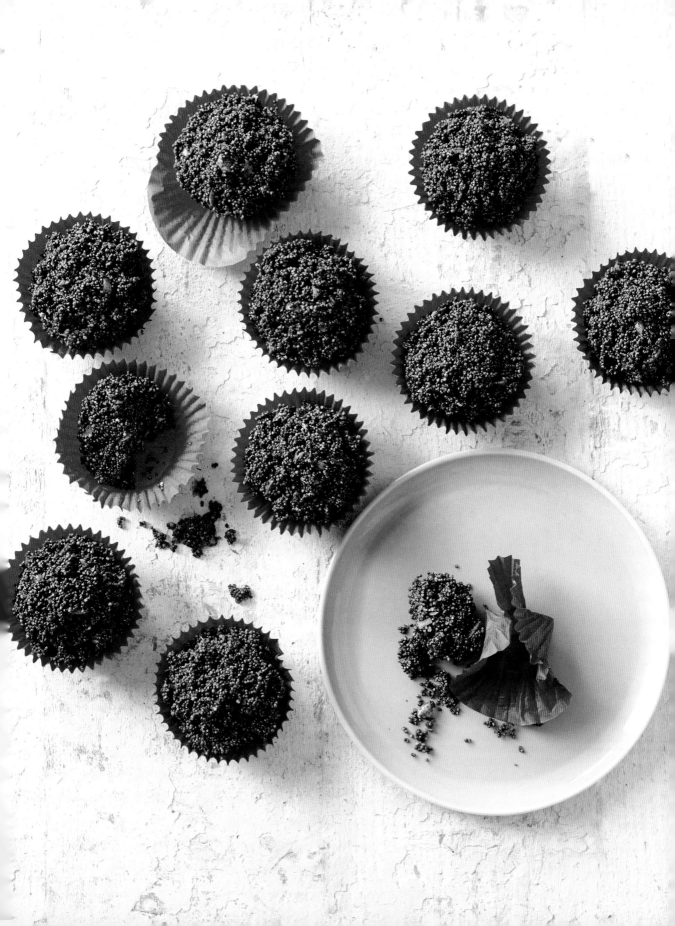

Nutter butter with banana

Preparation: 5 mins

Cooking time: nil

Serves: 2

Ingredients

2 brown rice cakes

1 tbsp cashew butter

1 banana, sliced

sprinkle of cinnamon

Method

Spread rice cakes with a thin layer of cashew butter. Arrange banana on top, sprinkle with cinnamon and enjoy!

MACRONUTRIENTS
per serve

Protein   4.2g   (0.1oz)

Fats   8.6g   (0.3oz)

Carbs   18.0g   (0.6oz)

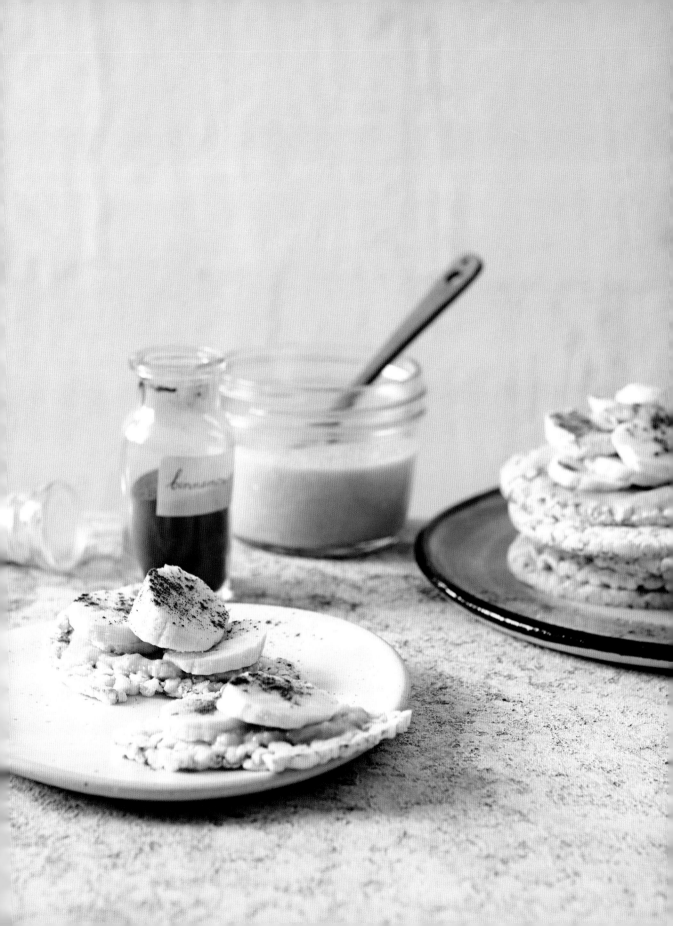

Protein parfait

Preparation: 10 mins

Cooking time: 20 mins (plus cooling time)

Serves: 2

Ingredients

300g (10.5oz) sheep's yoghurt

30 ml (1fl oz) agave nectar

1 tsp vanilla extract

20g (0.75oz) flaked almonds, toasted

20g (0.75oz) pumpkin seeds, toasted

20g (0.75oz) chia seeds

20g (0.75oz) flax seeds

½ tsp cinnamon

sprinkle of ground cloves

pinch of salt (iodised or Himalayan)

200g (7oz) mixed berries
(eg blueberries, raspberries, blackberries)

Method

In a medium bowl, whisk together the yoghurt, agave nectar and vanilla. Pour into a jug and set aside.

In another bowl, mix together the nuts, seeds and spices with a pinch of salt.

Set out two glasses. Pour in a little of the yoghurt, then layer with some of the seeds, some berries and then more yoghurt. Repeat with the remaining ingredients, cover with cling wrap and refrigerate until you're ready to eat.

MACRONUTRIENTS
per serve

Protein 13.8g (0.5oz)

Fats   21.2g (0.7oz)

Carbs   36.8g (1.3oz)

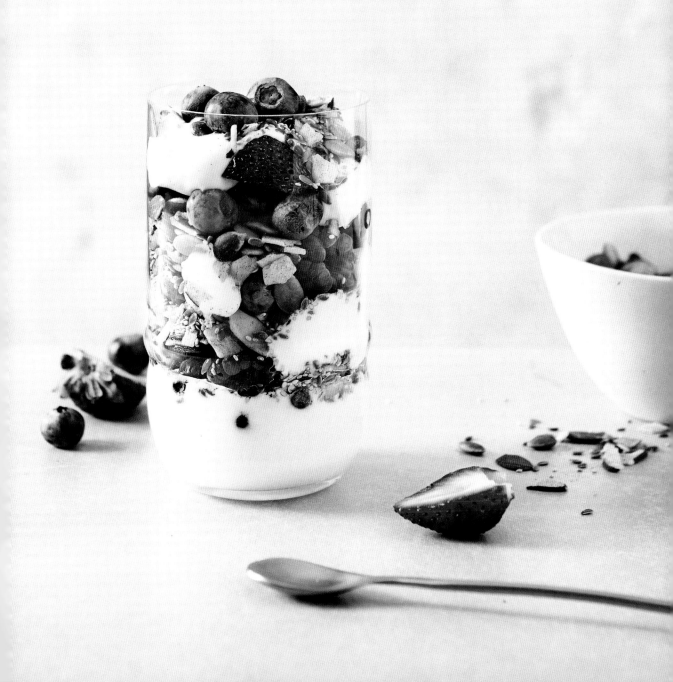

yours in health and fitness

Congratulations! Be proud of yourself for making it through my book, *Healthy body*. You are now an official shredder!

The principles within this book are designed to help you balance your hormones and create a body with less fat and more muscle tone – but they will also improve your mood and overall quality of life.

Remember, shredders, this is a lifestyle, not a diet. You have learned many new tools, but sometimes old habits can take time to break. Simply replace old habits that no longer serve you with better, healthier ones. You will feel better, look better and think more clearly. Everyone around you will be impressed with your new lean physique and also by a happier, healthier, more energetic you.

If you want to be fit and healthy, don't forget the following key principles to stay lean for life and keep those stubborn areas of body fat away.

- Protein is of utmost importance. Always ensure you have enough protein on your plate and throughout your day.
- Supplements will do exactly that – supplement – but nothing will substitute for good nutrition. There is no such thing as a magic pill but if you are diligent at following the recommendations, you will start to see stubborn areas of body fat melt away.
- Try to avoid, or at least cut down on, gluten and cow's milk for better digestion and less bloating. It will often take up to three months for the body to completely digest gluten, so it can take this long to see the effects of a gluten-free diet.
- Make your training part of your routine. Training at the same time every day is key if you struggle to stick to an exercise routine.
- Stay consistent. This is the only way you will see the results you seek. It gets easier to consistently choose the right lifestyle, but you have to start.
- Sometimes life gets busy and stressful. Don't beat yourself up if you fall off the wagon. My best piece of advice here is to jump straight back on and power ahead. We can all feel unmotivated at times and slip back into old habits, but the shorter the time you spend in your slump, the better you will bounce back and keep moving ahead.
- Documenting progress is also a motivating and important point, so keep a diary or journal. Take pictures so you know where you have come from and where you never want to go back to!

I would love to hear about your progress – email **info@sallymatterson.com.au** with your success stories and keep checking my website, **sallymatterson.com.au**, for updates.

Finally, don't forget that when you're fit, you're happy – you have the power within to begin your wellness journey. You can do it, shredders!

Yours in health and fitness,

Sally Matterson

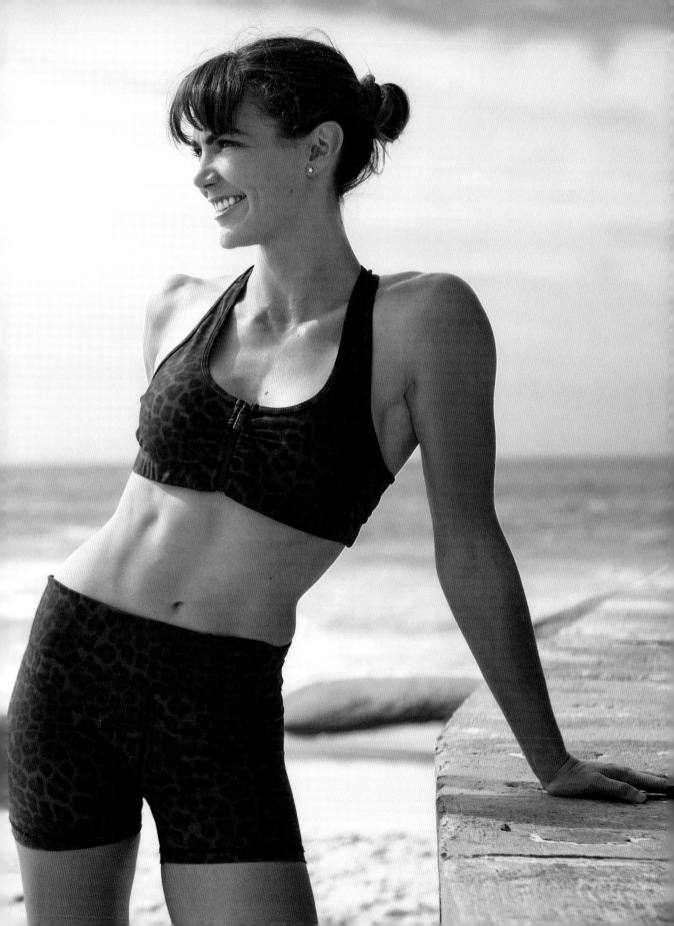

references

BOOKS

Bowden, J 2003, *Living the low-carb life: from Atkins to The Zone – choosing the diet that's right for you*, Sterling, New York.

Bowden, J 2007, *The 150 healthiest foods on earth: the surprising, unbiased truth about what you should eat and why*, Fair Winds Press, Vancouver.

Enig, MG 2000, *Know your fats: the complete primer for understanding the nutrition of fats, oils and cholesterol*, Bethesda Press, Maryland.

Poliquin, C 2013, Poliquin Group Education C 2013, Poliquin® BioSignature Modulation Course Notes, Poliquin Group, Rhode Island.

Poliquin, C 2006, *German body composition training manual*, Poliquin Group, Rhode Island.

Poliquin, C 2011, *Ask coach Poliquin*, Poliquin Group, Rhode Island.

ONLINE

Poliquin Group Editorial Staff 2010, 'HCL: the most important supplement ever?' <http://www.poliquingroup.com/ArticlesMultimedia/Articles/Article/433/HCLThe_Most_Important_Supplement_Ever.aspx> (downloaded 16 November 2014).

Poliquin Group Editorial Staff 2012, '10 ways to lower estrogen toxic load' <http://www.poliquingroup.com/articlesmultimedia/articles/article/801/10_ways_to_lower_estrogen_toxic_load_.aspx> (downloaded 16 November 2014).

Hines, S 2010, 'Biotyping is gaining popularity …' <http://www.ion.ac.uk/information/onarchives/autumnbiosignature-modulation-weight-loss-through-hormone-balance> (downloaded 16 November 2014).

index

L
L-carnitine 91
Liver 16, 17, 84, 85, 91, 92
Leucine 91
Love handles 12, 15
Lunge 30, 32, 40, 59, 61, 63, 79

M
Man boobs 17, 18, 82
Meal plans 22, 86, 87, 88, 89, 90
Medicine ball 22
Meditation 13
Menopause 15
Mental health 84
Menstruation 15
Metabolism 17, 19, 92
Minerals 17, 90, 92
Muffin top 15, 82
Multivitamin 17, 18, 90, 91

N
Naval 12, 13, 27
Nutrition 9, 12, 18, 22, 82

O
Obesity 18
Oestrogen (mimickers) 15, 16, 17, 18
Omega 3s 15, 19
Organic 16, 85

P
Pancreas 15
Paraben-free 16
Pear-shaped body 12, 15
Pesticides 16
Pharmacuetical-grade fish oil 15, 17, 18, 19, 91
Plastics 16
Poliquin 9
Practitioner 8, 9
Premenopausal 15
Probiotic 17
Protein powder 83, 144, 146, 148
Puperty 17
Push-ups 41, 57, 60, 67

Q
Quads 25, 26
Quinoa 106, 126, 144

R
Recipes 95
Reproduction 15
Results 9, 12
Row 27, 29

S
Serotonin 83, 84
Sex hormones 15, 18
Shoulder press 47
Skipping 13, 22, 39
Sleep 9, 13, 91
Sprinting 13
Squats 28, 39, 43
Stomach acid 17
Sugar 19, 85, 87
Suicide risk 13
Sulforaphane 16
Supplementation 9, 12, 16, 17, 18, 82, 91, 90, 92

T
Technique 22
Tempo 24
Testosterone 17, 18
Toning 17, 22, 25, 87
Toxins 8, 16
Triceps 67, 68, 69, 70

U
Upper chest fat 12, 17
Urine 17

V
Vitamin D 90
Vitamins 17, 90, 91, 92

W
Water 16, 93
Weight-bearing exercise 18, 22
Weight lifting 18
Weight loss 12
Weight plate 22
Wheat 84, 86
Workout 22, 23, 25

X
Xenoestrogens 16, 17

Z
Zinc (deficiency) 17, 18, 90